Underactive Bladder

Christopher R. Chapple
Alan J. Wein • Nadir I. Osman
Editors

Underactive Bladder

Springer

Editors
Christopher R. Chapple
Urology
The Royal Hallamshire Hospital
Sheffield
United Kingdom

Nadir I. Osman
Specialty Registrar
The Royal Hallamshire Hospital
Sheffield, South Yorkshire
United Kingdom

Alan J. Wein
West Pavilion, 3rd Floor
Urology, Perelman Center
Philadelphia, Pennsylvania
USA

ISBN 978-3-319-43085-0 ISBN 978-3-319-43087-4 (eBook)
DOI 10.1007/978-3-319-43087-4

Library of Congress Control Number: 2016957384

Printed on acid-free paper

This Springer imprint is published by Springer Nature
The registered company is Springer International Publishing AG Switzerland
The registered company is Gewerbestrasse 11, 6330 Cham, Switzerland

Contents

Contributors

Reem B. Aldamanhori, MD, MBBS, SB-Urol University Of Dammam, Khobar, Saudi Arabia

Royal Hallamshire Hospital, Sheffield, UK

K.E. Andersson, MD, PhD Institute for Regenerative Medicine, Wake Forest University, Winston Salem, NC, USA

Tim Boone, MD, PhD Department of Urology, Houston Methodist Hospital, Houston, TX, USA

C. R. Chapple Department of Urology, Royal Hallamshire Hospital, Sheffield, UK

Bilal Chughtai Department of Urology, Weill Cornell Medicine, New York, NY, USA

J. Drossaerts, MD Department of Urology, Maastricht University Medical Center, Maastricht, NL, The Netherlands

Christopher J. Hillary, MBChB, MRCS Academic Urology Unit, Royal Hallamshire Hospital, Sheffield, UK

R. Jairam, MD Department of Urology, Maastricht University Medical Center, Maastricht, NL, The Netherlands

Steven A. Kaplan, MD Icahn School of Medicine at Mount Sinai, New York, NY, USA

A. Kavanagh, MD Department of Urologic Sciences, University of British Columbia, Vancouver, BC, Canada

Philip E.V. Van Kerrebroeck, MD, PhD, MMSc Department of Urology, Maastricht University Medical Centre, Maastricht, The Netherlands

Gommert A. van Koeveringe, MD, PhD Department of Urology, Pelvic Care Center Maastricht, Maastricht UMC+, Maastricht, The Netherlands

Altaf Mangera, MBChB, FRCS, MD, FEBU Department of Urology, Sheffield Teaching Hospitals, Sheffield, UK

Nadir I. Osman Department of Urology, Royal Hallamshire Hospital, Sheffield, UK

Kevin L.J. Rademakers Maastricht University Medical Centre, Maastricht, The Netherlands

J. Stewart, MD Department of Urology, Houston Methodist Hospital, Houston, TX, USA

Austin Te Department of Urology, Weill Cornell Medicine, New York, NY, USA

Dominique Thomas Department of Urology, Weill Cornell Medicine, New York, NY, USA

A. J. Wein Urology, Perelman Center, Philadelphia, PA, USA

Introduction and Terminology

"I shall not attempt further to define the kinds of material I understand to be embraced within that shorthand description and perhaps I could never succeed in intelligibly doing so. But I do know it when I see it, and the motion picture involved in this case is not that." Thus concluded a statement by Justice Potter Stewart of the United States Supreme Court in 1964 when offering an opinion in the case of Jacovellis vs The State of Ohio. The appellant, Jacovellis, the manager of a motion picture theatre, was convicted under a state obscenity law of possessing and exhibiting an allegedly obscene film, "Les Amants," and the state supreme court upheld the conviction. The conviction was reversed by the United States Supreme Court which held that the film was not obscene under the applicable standards. Wikipedia accurately categorizes the phrase "I know it when I see it" as "a colloquial expression by which a speaker attempts to categorize an observable fact or event, although the category is subjective or lacks clearly defined parameters." Unfortunately, this is precisely the case with "the underactive bladder (UAB)" and "detrusor underactivity (DU)." The phrase "underactive bladder" carries more of a symptomatic implication, whereas "detrusor underactivity" implies a urodynamic finding or set of findings.

Detrusor underactivity has also been described in the literature as detrusor hypotonicity, impaired detrusor contractility, detrusor failure, acontractile detrusor or, simply, a poorly contracting detrusor. The current "official" International Continence Society (ICS) definition of detrusor underactivity is "a contraction of reduced strength or duration resulting in prolonged bladder emptying and/or a failure to achieve complete bladder emptying within a normal time span" [1]. On the surface, this sounds very erudite and the result of a prolonged committee meeting or many such meetings. The problem of course is that there is no specific definition of any of the following descriptive terms:

Reduced strength
Reduced duration
Prolonged
Complete bladder emptying
Normal time span

Acontractile detrusor is defined as one that cannot be demonstrated to contract during urodynamic studies.

Ideally, UAB should be a clinical condition characterized by symptoms which may be bothersome or nonbothersome, but also by specific agreed-upon objective urodynamic measurements. The situation is a little different from the relationship between overactive bladder and detrusor overactivity. Clearly, the symptom syndrome of overactive bladder (urgency with or without urgency incontinence usually with frequency and nocturia in the absence of infection or other obvious pathologies) can exist without detrusor overactivity. The term urgency, the main requirement of overactive bladder, has a very specific definition, as does detrusor overactivity (an involuntary bladder contraction during the filling phase which may be spontaneous or provoked). There is no specific consensus-based definition of UAB, and the same situation applies to DU. The ideal state of affairs would be to have a specific set of symptoms (or at least one symptom – similar to urgency) that would characterize UAB and have a set of measurements or a measurement that would be agreed upon to characterize DU. Ideally, these symptoms/measurements should be able to be characterized in such a way that a score or scale of severity, accepted by clinicians and regulators, could be formulated and used to judge improvement, worsening, or stability.

The ideal situation would be to be able to quantitatively characterize DU urodynamically and then relate these measurements to a group of symptoms whose presence would then suggest the urodynamic entity. Unfortunately, the commonly used noninvasive parameters of residual urine volume and peak and mean flow rate are factors which simply integrate the activity of the bladder and the outlet during the emptying phase of micturition, and thus it is impossible to discern whether abnormally low flow rates or high residual urine volumes are due to a problem with the bladder, the outlet, or both. There are a number of "contraction parameters," the most commonly used of which is the bladder contractility index (BCI), which gives approximately the same information regarding detrusor contraction strength as the Schaefer nomogram [2–4]. The formula Pdet@Qmax+5Qmax characterizes contractility as very weak (equal to or greater than 50), weak (50–100), normal (100–150), and strong (equal to or greater than 150). However, this is applicable only to men, does not measure the sustainability of contraction, and is dependent on the degree of urethral resistance which of course differs from one patient to another. Osman et al. [5] summarized the methods for assessing detrusor contractility and described the Watts factor [6] as a measurement which is minimally dependent on the volume of urine and one that is not affected by the presence of bladder outlet obstruction. However, more recently published data have appeared showing that the Wmax as well as the BCI continually rise with an increasing grade of obstruction [7, 8] and propose a new nomogram for simultaneous classification of bladder outlet obstruction and bladder contractility. Additionally, they propose and cite prior evidence that in men detrusor wall thickness determined by suprapubic ultrasound of equal to or greater than 1.23 mm in combination with a bladder capacity of greater than 445 ml can sufficiently predict detrusor underactivity in men. Quite relevant in these articles is the suggestion that what is really necessary is a methodology to accurately access the compensatory capacity of detrusor contractility and the contractile reserve, and also the capacity of the outlet to relax. In discussing the prevalence of DU in patients with nonneurogenic lower urinary tract symptoms, Osman et al. [5] list nine different published urodynamic definitions for men and four qualitative and two quantitative definitions for women. Thus, it would seem that an accepted definition of detrusor underactivity has yet to be agreed upon, with obviously, different parameters for at least age and gender.

The original ICS definition of DU was in effect a qualitative urodynamic definition, but was meant to suggest a certain pattern of symptomatology. The joint report (IUGA/ICS) on the Terminology for Female Pelvic Floor Dysfunction [9] did not change the definition of either detrusor underactivity or acontractile detrusor. Smith et al. [10] in a report resulting from a 2014 International Consultation on Incontinence-Research Society (ICI-RS) think tank, not published until 2 years later, pointed out that the formal definition of DU was descriptive of a relative dysfunction and contained no stipulation of symptoms or etiology. They verbalized current thinking by stating that the diagnosis of DU suggested a "likely symptom complex characterized by impaired voiding, including poor and/or intermittent stream, sensations of incomplete empting, double voiding, and possibly hesitancy and terminal dribbling." In concluding their article, they describe the patient experience of UAB as "the symptom complex of prolonged urination, with or without a sensation of incomplete bladder emptying, usually with hesitancy and a slow stream." They pointed out that this definition was based strictly on expert opinion and that a formal definition of UAB should be developed, based on patient experience. The problem of course is that the symptoms of decreased stream, hesitancy, feeling of incomplete emptying, and interrupted stream are shared by men and women alike with DU, bladder outlet obstruction and are present in some normal individuals as well.

A consensus group was formed by Chris Chapple under the auspices of the ICS to deal with terminology relative to UAB/DU, and their initial working definition for the symptom complex that they called underactive bladder, a term which suggests detrusor underactivity but is not synonymous with it (an analogy to the relationship between the term overactive bladder symptom syndrome and the urodynamic finding of detrusor overactivity) was, "The underactive bladder is a symptom complex suggestive of detrusor underactivity and is usually characterized by prolonged urination time with or without a sensation of incomplete bladder emptying, usually with hesitancy, reduced sensation on filling and a slow stream" [11]. A later symptomatic definition from this consensus committee was slightly different: "Lower urinary tract symptoms are not disease specific. The symptoms of hesitancy, straining to void and a slow stream can be characteristic of both outflow obstruction and detrusor underactivity. The underactive bladder is characterized by hesitancy, a feeling of incomplete bladder emptying and a reduced sensation of filling of the bladder with or without leakage or night time frequency." As of the time of the writing of this chapter, the proposed definition of the committee, now titled as a standardization subcommittee of the ICS, is as follows: "Underactive bladder is characterized by a slow urinary stream, hesitancy and straining to void, with or without a feeling of incomplete bladder emptying and dribbling, often with storage symptoms." Footnotes add "underactive bladder occurs in association with diverse pathophysiologies and based on current knowledge there is no single distinguishing symptom" and "storage symptoms are varied and maybe highly prevalent, including nocturia, increased daytime frequency, reduced sensation of filling and incontinence. Underlying mechanisms of storage symptoms are diverse and are often related to a significant post voiding residual urine volume."

Are there symptoms which typify DU and could therefore be used in an evidence-based definition of UAB? Most published work until recently would argue that the symptoms are shared by those attributable to bladder outlet obstruction [5, 11], dysfunctional voiding [7] and many of these symptoms, though not in the aggregate, are voiced by individuals without significant lower urinary tract dysfunction.

Recently, Gammie et al. [12] reported on the analysis of 28 years of urodynamic data from a single center to identify clinical predictors of detrusor underactivity on urodynamic study, particularly in comparison to bladder outlet obstruction. They concluded that there are signs and symptoms that can distinguish patients with DU from those with normal pressure flow studies and from patients with bladder outlet obstruction. At the outset, they established concrete criteria for bladder contractility index, bladder outlet obstruction index, percent of bladder voiding efficiency for what they described as detrusor underactivity, bladder outlet obstruction, and "normal" pressure flow studies for both men and women. These were age adjusted. Though a positive odds ratio existed for many symptoms and historical factors, rarely was any one exclusive to one of the three groups. The ones that were, were of low frequency. For instance, the symptom of decreased urinary stream in men was reported by 56 % of those with DU, 82 % of those with BOO, and 30 % of normal patients. The numbers for hesitancy were 51, 69, and 26 % and for feeling of incomplete emptying, 36, 29, and 22 %. On the other hand, absent or decreased sensation was reported by 13 % of men with DU, 0 % with BOO, and 3 % of those with normal pressure flow parameters. For women, the symptom of decreased stream was reported by 29 % of those with DU, 20 % of those with BOO, and 4 % of individuals with normal PFS. The percents for hesitancy were 28, 27, and 9.1 %, for feeling of incomplete emptying 28, 36, and 20 %. Absent or decreased sensation was reported by 4.3, 0, and 0.8 %. The dividing lines still seem blurred.

Finally, one could divide UAB broadly into neurogenic and myogenic. It remains to be seen whether this distinction would be useful in terms of symptomatology, urodynamics, or therapy. Neurogenic implies that myocyte and detrusor contractility are intact and that insufficiencies in expulsive pressure efforts result from inadequate stimulation once the micturition reflex is triggered [10]. The myocyte hypothesis implies either a cellular (muscle cell) dysfunction and/or a whole organ deficiency.

So, in summary at the outset of this book on UAB and therefore DU, virtually all would agree with the following statement: we have a common condition that we think we can recognize, yet cannot define or quantitate, which often is a contributory factor in failure to empty and in common lower urinary tract symptoms but with no agreed upon indications for treatment, except for urinary retention, and no established agreed upon routinely successful therapy. The introduction began with one applicable quote, it will close with another that seems relevant to the topics, "The more one knows, the more one knows how little one knows…the less one understands, the less one understands how little one knows" [13].

Alan J. Wein and Christopher R. Chapple

References

1. Abrams P, Cardozo L, Fall M, et al. The standardization of terminology of lower urinary tract function. Neurourol Urodyn. 2002;21:167–78.
2. Schaefer W. Basic principles and advanced analysis of bladder voiding function. Urol Clin N Am. 1990;17:533–66.
3. Schäfer W. Analysis of bladder-outlet function with the linearized passive urethral resistance relation, linPURR, and a disease-specific approach for grading obstruction: from complex to simple. World J Urol. 1995;13:47–58.
4. Abrams P. Bladder outlet obstruction index, bladder contractility index and bladder voiding efficiency: three simple indices to define bladder voiding function. BJU Int. 1999;84:14–15.
5. Osman N, Chapple C, Abrams P, et al. Detrusor underactivity and the underactive bladder: a new clinical entity? A review of current terminology, definitions, epidemiology, aetiology, and diagnosis. Eur Urol. 2014;65:389–98.
6. Griffiths D. Assessment of detrusor contraction strength or contractility. Neurourol Urodyn. 1991;10:1–18.
7. Van Koeveringe G, Rademakers K. Factors impacting bladder underactivity and clinical implications. Minerva Urol Nefrol. 2015;67:139–48.
8. Rademakers K, Van Koeveringe G, Oelke M. Detrusor underactivity in men with lower urinary tract symptoms/benign prostatic obstruction: characterization and potential impact on indications for surgical treatment of the prostate. Curr Opin Urol. 2016;26:3–10.
9. Haylen B, de Ridder D, Freeman R, et al. An International Urogynecological Association (IUGA)/International Continence Society (ICS) joint report on the terminology for female pelvic floor dysfunction. Neurourol Urodyn (2010);29:4–20
10. Smith P, Birder L, Abrams P, Wein A, Chapple C. Detrusor underactivity and the underactive bladder: Symptoms, function, cause-what do we mean? ICI-RS think tank 2014. Neurourol Urodyn. 2016;35:312–7.
11. Chapple C, Osman N, Birder L, et al. The underactive bladder: a new clinical concept? Eur Urol. 2015;68:351–3.
12. Gammie A, Kaper M, Dorrepaal C, et al. Signs and symptoms of detrusor underactivity: an analysis of clinical presentation and urodynamic tests from a large group of patients undergoing pressure-flow studies. Eur Urol. 2016;69:361–9.
13. Turner-Warwick R, Chapple C. Functional reconstruction of the urinary tract and gynaeco-urology. Oxford: Blackwell Publishing; 2002. p. 1.

Pathophysiology and Associations of Underactive Bladder

1

K.E. Andersson

Key Points

- Underactive bladder (UAB) and detrusor underactivity (DUA) are common, aging-related, multifactorial conditions
- Aging may be an etiological factor, but concomitant disorders may aggravate aging-induced reduction in bladder structure and function
- Bladder outflow obstruction, diabetes mellitus, neurogenic disorders, and ischemic bladder dysfunction, are often associated with UAB/DUA
- Impaired detrusor contractility has been regarded as a major etiologic factor of UAB/DUA, but disturbances of bladder sensory afferents and the central nervous system control of micturition and changes in efferent neurotransmission may be as important
- Chronic bladder ischemia and resultant oxidative stress may cause detrusor overactivity progressing to DUA and inability to empty the bladder.

Introduction

Impaired bladder emptying is a common clinical condition described in different ways. Detrusor underactivity (DU or DUA) has been defined by the International Continence Society [1] and is a urodynamic diagnosis requiring invasive pressure flow studies (PFS). It is defined as a detrusor contraction of reduced strength and/or

K.E. Andersson, MD, PhD
Institute for Regenerative Medicine, Wake Forest University School of Medicine, Winston Salem, NC, USA

Clinical Medicine, Department of Obstetrics and Gynecology, Aarhus University Hospital, Palle Juul-Jensens Boulevard 99, DK 8200 Aarhus N, Denmark
e-mail: karl-erik.andersson@med.lu.se

C.R. Chapple et al. (eds.), *Underactive Bladder*,
DOI 10.1007/978-3-319-43087-4_1

duration, resulting in prolonged bladder emptying and/or a failure to achieve complete bladder emptying within a normal time span. It is characterized by a low-pressure, poorly sustained, or wave-like detrusor contraction with an associated poor flow rate [2, 3]. In order to identify the clinical features associated with DUA, Gammie et al. [3] investigated 1788 patient records (men: 507; women: 1281) classified as DUA, bladder outflow obstruction (BOO), or normal PFS. They found that both men and women with DUA reported a statistically significantly higher occurrence of decreased and/or interrupted urinary stream, hesitancy, feeling of incomplete bladder emptying, palpable bladder, feeling of incomplete bowel emptying, absent and/or decreased sensation, and always straining to void, compared with men and women with normal PFS. However, Gammie et al. [3] also found interesting differences between the groups and concluded that there are signs and symptoms that can distinguish men and women with DUA from patients with normal PFS, and further distinguish between DUA and BOO.

The term underactive bladder (UAB) has been used by several investigators [4, 5] referring to a clinical condition in a broader sense mirroring the overactive bladder (OAB) syndrome. Based on their findings, Gammie et al. [3] concluded that the clinical presentation of DUA patients is consistent with the UAB working definition suggested by Osman et al. [5] and "justifies developing and testing a diagnostic algorithm based on the signs and symptoms of DUA."

The causes of UAB/DUA can be classified in different ways dependent on associated morbidities [6–10]. UAB/DUA can involve a spectrum of pathophysiologically different mechanisms e.g., the central nervous system (CNS) control, sensory functions, detrusor neurotransmission and smooth muscle activity [6–10], and disturbances of any of these components can result in reduced ability to empty the bladder. However, more than one pathophysiological mechanism can be involved in the symptoms and urodynamic manifestations in an individual patient. Since in many cases UAB/DUA is associated with and/or may be the result of a known morbidity, a clinically meaningful way to describe the disorder could be e.g., UAB/DUA associated with diabetes, and then (when possible) further define the major mechanisms involved. For example, is the condition a result of myogenic changes, such as loss of muscle tissue and increased collagen deposition – reduced contractile strength?; are the motor nerves involved – defective neurotransmission?; are bladder afferent nerves or CNS control involved – reduced sensation? Since pharmacologic treatment based on targeting specific mechanisms, e.g., muscarinic receptors has not been successful, the combination of treatment focusing not only on the bladder condition, but also on specific factors related to the associated morbidity may increase the treatment success rate. For example, many new disease-modifying drugs have been approved and introduced for treatment of multiple sclerosis (MS). These drugs may have effects not only on the MS disease process, but also on the disease symptoms, including UAB/DUA [6, 10].

The present overview is an update with focus on some morbidities often associated with UAB/DUA, i.e., aging, bladder outflow obstruction, diabetes mellitus, neurogenic disorders, and ischemic bladder dysfunction.

Common Associations of UAB/DUA

UAB/DUA is commonly occurring and several aspects of the condition have been discussed in recent excellent reviews [7–9, 11–14]. Many different diseases/disorders can be associated with UAB/DUA and these may either be a direct cause of the bladder condition, or a contributing factor to another independent process e.g., aging. Even though there are abundant reviews on the causes/mechanisms of UAB/DUA, there is a lack of original studies on this condition focusing specifically on underlying morbidities.

Ageing

Aging is a normal process, but a spectrum of changes occurs in the lower urinary tract (LUT) with increasing age, and it seems that some changes occur in everyone if they live long enough. However, UAB/DUA can hardly be considered as a consequence of the progression of normal aging. Current evidence clearly indicates that impaired voiding function has an age-associated prevalence [15]. However, figures on prevalence are dependent on the population investigated, and what is defined as impaired voiding. In 85 ambulatory, non-demented, community-dwelling female volunteers, stratified into age groups 20–39 (n-19), 40–59 (n=30), and>60 (n=36) years, Pfisterer et al. [16] found that most elderly individuals continued to empty their bladder almost completely, with normal voiding frequency. Urodynamically, urethral closure pressure, detrusor contraction strength, and urine flow rate declined significantly with age, regardless of whether DO was present. Bladder capacity did not decrease with age, but, as could be expected, was smaller in subjects with DO. Surprisingly, despite the fact that the proportion of urine excreted at night was found to increase significantly with age, the mean number of nocturnal voids was less than one in all age groups. Importantly, bladder sensation diminished significantly with age, but was stronger in subjects with DO. A reduction of bladder sensation with age was also found by Collas and Malone-Lee [17] based on results from urodynamic investigation of 1381 women (age range 20–95 years, mean 54.9) with symptoms of LUT dysfunction.

Age-related impairment in detrusor contractility has been regarded as a major etiologic factor of UAB/DUA. However, results are conflicting. Karram et al. [18] found that maximal detrusor pressure did not correlate with age in a study comparing 30 healthy asymptomatic female volunteers to 70 women with stress urinary incontinence, and Madersbacher et al. [19] observed no age related changes in maximum detrusor pressure or $p_{det.Qmax}$ in 436 patients (253 men and 183 women) aged >40 years referred with LUT symptoms (LUTS). Ameda et al. [20] performed video urodynamic studies of 193 symptomatic men without outlet obstruction (31 % having impaired contractility and 11 % detrusor instability and impaired contractility). They found that bladder contractility did not correlate with age. Malone-Lee and Wahedna [21] described age-related changes in detrusor muscle function using urodynamic data obtained from 1391 women and 324 men. They found that older patients of both sexes had higher residual urine volumes. There were no age-related differences in isometric detrusor function, but older women showed lower detrusor shortening velocities. Valentini et al. [22] studied a group of 449 women with LUTS referred for urodynamic investigation. They were stratified into three groups; age 55–64, 65–74 and 75–93 years. In the oldest age group maximal detrusor pressure, $p_{det.Qmax}$ and flow rate declined in those without DO. Zimmern et al. [23] investigating two large cohorts of women (age range 27–75 years) planning stress urinary incontinence (SUI) surgery, found that hypocontractility was more likely in women ≥65 years, and their main conclusion was that detrusor contractility and efficiency decrease with age. In 1,179 patients aged over 65 years, who had undergone a urodynamic study for LUTS and having no neurological or anatomical conditions [24], 40.2 % of men and 13.3 % of women were classified as having DU, and there was an age-related increase in prevalence. In men, the prevalence of bladder outflow obstruction (BOO) was constant across the age spectrum, but the prevalence of DUA and DO increased with age, and 46.5 % of men with DUA also had DO or BOO. In women, the prevalence of DUA also increased with age, and the trend was more remarkable in women aged over 70 years.

Whether or not a decrease of detrusor contractility is a primary contributor to age-related impairment of bladder emptying has not been conclusively demonstrated [25]. Since there are several limitations of all the clinical studies referred to, definitive conclusions on the importance of detrusor contractility are uncertain, and it has been suggested that *in vitro* studies on human detrusor muscle are required [8]. In isolated human bladder preparations obtained from biopsies (n = 227) of four different groups of patients: stable bladders (control), bladder outlet obstruction, idiopathic, and neurogenic DO, there was no evidence for a decline of detrusor smooth muscle contractility or excitability as a function of age, nor any gender difference or presence of pathology. However, in the pathology groups there was evidence for a decline of functional innervation with age [26]. Even if these findings do not exclude an age-related decrease of detrusor contractility as an important factor in the pathogenesis of UAB, they suggest that other factors may be as important as this parameter.

Bladder Outflow Obstruction

In men with BOO, impaired detrusor contractility has been regarded as the most common cause of UAB/DUA in older men. However, its importance in age-related voiding dysfunction is unclear [25], and there is evidence suggesting that detrusor contractility does not decline in patients with long-term BOO. Based on repeat pressure–flow urodynamic studies in 196 men with bladder outlet obstruction (with a minimum 10-year gap from the first assessment), Al-Hayek et al. [27] found no evidence to suggest that detrusor contractility declines with long-term BOO. Relieving the obstruction surgically did not improve the contractility. It was also found that underactive detrusors remained underactive but did not get worse with time, and the authors suggested that this could indicate that the aging process per se does not lead to UAB/DUA. BOO is uncommon in elderly women, nevertheless, Arbarbanel and Marcus [28] detected impaired detrusor contractility (IDC), defined as Pdet at Qmax < 30cmH$_2$O and Qmax < 10 ml, in 12 (12 %) of 99 women 70 years old or older with storage and/or voiding LUTS who had undergone urodynamic pressure-flow studies in a urodynamic referral center during a 2-year period.

Since it is well established that BOO can result in chronic changes within the bladder wall that may predispose to the UAB/DUA [29–31], it is reasonable to consider BOO *per se* as a potential cause of UAB/DUA, but also as contributory factor in the development of aging-related UAB/DUA.

Diabetes Mellitus

Diabetic voiding dysfunction (DVD) seems to be a far more common complication of DM than commonly recognized and has been observed in 80 % of individuals with DM complications. By comparison, neuropathy and nephropathy have been reported to affect 60 % and 50 % of diabetic patients, respectively [32]. Many studies have revealed that diabetes mellitus (DM) can be associated with a wide range of LUT dysfunctions (for reviews, see [32–36]). The term diabetic cystopathy was introduced by Frimodt-Moller [37, 38] more or less as an end-stage disorder which was characterized by irreversible loss of sensation developing into a distended bladder with a high risk of urinary retention. Persistent overdistension of the bladder was believed to gradually cause impaired detrusor contraction. However, the term diabetic cystopathy is now often used synonymously with diabetic voiding dysfunction (DVD) with varying symptoms including OAB, impaired sensation of bladder fullness, increased bladder capacity, reduced bladder contractility, increased residual urine, and UAB/DUA. Moreover, common concomitant diseases such as urinary tract infection, benign prostatic hyperplasia (BPH), and stress urinary incontinence may obscure underlying DVD. Many studies have shown that DM can be associated with a time-dependent decline in voiding efficiency over the course of the disease [39, 40]. Increasing epidemiologic evidence suggests that diabetes significantly increases the risks of BPH and LUTS [41, 42].

The pathophysiology of DM associated DVD/UAB/DU is considered multifactorial, involving neuronal, smooth muscle, and urothelial dysfunction [40]. Therefore, it is important to discern the major factor from the complex presentation of symptoms that can be observed in an individual patient. It has also been reported that DVD/diabetic cystopathy can occur silently and early in the course of DM. In those cases, it is typical that bladder dysfunction induced by DM is only found with careful questioning and/or urodynamic testing.

It is well established that hyperglycemia is the main driver of diabetic complications and mainly responsible for the autonomic neuropathy causing DVD and eventually UAB/DUA [43, 44]. Its deleterious effects are attributable, among other things, to the formation advanced glycation end products (AGEs), ischemia, superoxide-induced free-radical formation, and impaired axonal transport [40]. An involvement of nerve growth factor (NGF) has been suggested based on animal experiments [45], but its role in humans is unclear.

Strategies to achieve optimal glycaemic control such as diet, exercise and weight loss have been recommended as a means to stop progression of the structural and functional changes occurring in DM [40]. DM is a systemic disease involving not only the genitourinary system, but also other visceral structures, including the cardiovascular and gastrointestinal systems. Treatment of disturbances in these systems may benefit also the LUT.

Neurogenic Disorders

Neurologic disorders, injury to the spinal cord, cauda equina and pelvic plexus, and infectious neurologic problems may all cause UAB/DUA [12]. Other common disorders associated with UAB/DUA are stroke, Parkinson's disease and multiple sclerosis (MS).

Stroke After stroke, urinary incontinence occurs with a prevalence ranging from 37 to 79 % in the acute phase. One year after stroke, approximately one-third of patients remain incontinent [46, 47]. Urinary retention is common in the acute phase and within 72 h following a stroke approximately 50 % of patients had urinary retention, mainly due to detrusor areflexia, as demonstrated by urodynamic evaluations [48, 49]. However, 95 % of these patients will resume voiding within 2 months after the incident [50].

It is generally accepted that the most common urodynamic finding in stroke patients is DO. Thus, Pizzi et al. [47] found DO in 56 %, DO with impaired contractility (DOIC) in 14 %, and DUA in 15 % of 106 stroke patients immediately after admission. After 1 month urodynamic studies, repeated on 63 patients, showed normal results in 30 %, DO in 48 %, DOIC in 6 %, and DUA in 16 %. Attempts to correlate the type of stroke (hemorrhagic and ischemic) or location of lesion with the type of bladder dysfunction have given diverging results [48, 50–53].

As pointed out by Kadow et al. [12] an important point to consider in evaluating stroke patients is that they often have other comorbidities, such as DM or prior neurologic diseases, and that this history can contribute to their bladder dysfunction.

Parkinson's disease Disturbances of lower urinary tract function are frequently observed in sufferers of Parkinson's disease (PD), and in the literature storage symptoms have been reported to be present in 57–83 % of patients, whereas voiding symptoms can be observed in 17–27 % [54]. In different studies the reported occurrence of UAB/DUA varies. Thus, Araki et al. [55] found DUA (hyporeflexia or areflexia) in 11 out 70 (16 %) PD patients assessed urodynamically, whereas Uchiyama et al. [56] investigating 50 consecutive untreated PD patients, found that 64 % complained of urinary symptoms (storage, 64.0 %; voiding, 28.0 %). Abnormal findings in the storage phase were found in in 84 %, with DO and increased bladder sensation without DO in 58.0 % and 12.0 % of patients, respectively. In the voiding phase, DUA, impaired urethral relaxation such as detrusor sphincter dyssynergia (DSD), and bladder outlet obstruction were present in 50.0 %, 8.0 % and 16 % of patients, respectively. In patients with both storage and voiding phase abnormalities, DO + DUA was the most common finding. Liu et al. [57] found DUA in 53 % of 58 patients investigated urodynamically.

The pathophysiology underlying DUA in PD is currently not well understood [58], but is thought to reflect an altered frontal–basal ganglia circuit [57]. Overall motor impairment was found significantly related to detrusor weakness but not to DO [57]. Both dyssynergia of the EUS during neurogenic DO and bradykinesia of the EUS during the onset of voluntary micturition can occur in PD patients [58]. Both of these EUS abnormalities can lead to impaired detrusor contractility and DUA.

Many patients initially diagnosed with PD may have Multiple System Atrophy (MSA), and it is important to distinguish the two as their urological management is different.

Multiple sclerosis A majority of patients diagnosed with multiple sclerosis (MS) will develop LUTS during the course of the disease and urologic problems are reported in up to 75 % of patients [59]. Symptoms most often result from involvement of the spinal cord, which results in DO and DSD. LUT symptoms may change with time, paralleling the dynamic course of MS [60]. MS patients may present with both storage and voiding symptoms, and urodynamic studies have shown that the most prevalent urinary conditions in these patients are DO, DSD, and detrusor hypocontractility [60–64]. Litwiller et al. [64] reviewed 22 published series of primarily symptomatic MS patients (total N = 1882), and found neurogenic DO present in 62 % of patients as the primary urodynamic diagnosis; DSD occurred in 25 % and hypocontractility in 20 % of patients. However, most MS patients have a combination of these urological conditions. Amarenco et al. [65] investigated 65 patients suffering from MS and presenting with urological dysfunction. Forty-five (69 %) patients suffered from overactive bladder, 48 (73 %) from voiding dysfunction, and 14 (21 %) from urinary retention. Urodynamic investigation demonstrated DO in 46 (70 %) cases, and DUA in four (6 %) cases.

The location of the neurologic lesion plays a critical role in the type of resultant bladder dysfunction. Araki et al. [66] that patients with cervical cord lesions or pontine lesions are more likely to suffer from emptying symptoms, including DUA, whereas those with cerebral cortex lesions are more prone to storage symptoms such as DO. Medullary lesions between the pontine and sacral micturition centres were reported to cause urethral dysfunction, with DSD being the most extreme defect [64]. Typical symptoms suggestive of DSD in these patients are hesitancy, intermittent stream and a high post-void residual (PVR) [62].

Ischemic Bladder Disease

Vascular endothelial dysfunction and urological symptoms are common in e.g., the metabolic syndrome, and occur also during the human aging process, and the vascular changes are an independent risk factor for the development of atherosclerosis and hypertension [67]. Pelvic arterial insufficiency may lead to impaired lower urinary tract perfusion and play an important role in the development of bladder dysfunction such as DO and the OAB syndrome [68–71]. It has been suggested [72], and has been shown in animal experiments [73] that chronic ischemia-related bladder dysfunction may progress to UAB/DUA. It is desirable to treat not only symptoms, but also the progression of the morphological bladder changes induced by chronic ischemia. Studies in experimental models in rabbits and rats have shown that pelvic arterial insufficiency may result in significant bladder ischemia with reduced bladder wall oxygen tension [74–77]. In turn, this will lead to oxidative stress associated with upregulation of oxidative stress sensitive genes, increased muscarinic receptor activity, ultrastructural damage, and neurodegeneration [76–79]. It has also been shown in rabbits that moderate ischemia causes DO, whereas severe ischemia causes DUA [74]. In an established rat model where chronic bladder ischemia was induced by iliac arterial injury + high cholesterol diet for 8 weeks, neointimal formation, luminal occlusion and bladder ischemia could be demonstrated [76, 77]. Urodynamically, micturition intervals were significantly decreased and bladder capacity and voided volume significantly lower than in controls. In vitro, contractile responses of bladder strips to KCl, electrical field stimulation and carbachol were significantly less than in controls. Bladders from the arterial injury animals also showed a significantly increased percentage of collagen.

Several types of drug may be able to prevent some of these changes. Even if the PDE5 inhibitor tadalafil [80], the α1-adrenoceptor (AR) blocker, silodosin [81], the β_3-AR agonist mirabegron [82], and the free radical scavenger, melatonin [80, 83], were unable to prevent the development of neo-intimal hyperplasia and bladder ischemia, they all exerted a protecting effect on urodynamic parameters, and on the functional and morphological changes of the bladder demonstrable in vitro. The different mechanisms of action of the different drugs suggest a multifactorial pathogenesis of chronic ischemia-induced bladder dysfunction. Since several of the agents tested are used clinically for relieving LUTS, the results from the animal models seem to have translational value, and may be of relevance for designing clinical studies to demonstrate if the drugs may prevent progression of ischemia-related functional and morphological bladder changes.

Summary and Future Directions

Impaired bladder emptying is a common clinical condition, which may be associated by a variety of morbidities and a spectrum of pathophysiologically different mechanisms. In order to understand UAB/DUA identification of the underlying cause(s) is necessary either by clinical symptoms or by e.g., urodynamics. Effective pharmacologic therapy is lacking, but combining individually designed standard therapy with optimized treatment of associated co-morbidities may lead to improved outcomes.

References

1. Abrams P, Cardozo L, Fall M, Griffiths D, Rosier P, Ulmsten U, van Kerrebroeck P, Victor A, Wein A. The standardisation of terminology of lower urinary tract function: report from the Standardisation Sub-committee of the International Continence Society. Neurourol Urodyn. 2002;21(2):167–78.
2. Thomas AW, Cannon A, Bartlett E, Ellis-Jones J, Abrams P. The natural history of lower urinary tract dysfunction in men: the influence of detrusor underactivity on the outcome after transurethral resection of the prostate with a minimum 10-year urodynamic follow-up. BJU Int. 2004;93(6):745–50.
3. Gammie A, Kaper M, Dorrepaal C, Kos T, Abrams P. Signs and symptoms of detrusor underactivity: an analysis of clinical presentation and urodynamic tests from a large group of patients undergoing pressure flow studies. Eur Urol. 2016;69(2):361–9.
4. Miyazato M, Yoshimura N, Chancellor MB. The other bladder syndrome: underactive bladder. Rev Urol. 2013;15(1):11–22.
5. Osman NI, Chapple CR, Abrams P, Dmochowski R, Haab F, Nitti V, Koelbl H, van Kerrebroeck P, Wein AJ. Detrusor underactivity and the underactive bladder–a new clinical entity? A review of current terminology, definitions, epidemiology, aetiology and diagnosis. Eur Urol. 2014;65(2):389–98.
6. Andersson KE. The many faces of impaired bladder emptying. Curr Opin Urol. 2014;24(4): 363–9.
7. Drake MJ, Williams J, Bijos DA. Voiding dysfunction due to detrusor underactivity: an overview. Nat Rev Urol. 2014;11(8):454–64.
8. Osman NI, Chapple CR. Contemporary concepts in the aetiopathogenesis of detrusor underactivity. Nat Rev Urol. 2014;11(11):639–48.
9. Yoshida M, Yamaguchi O. Detrusor underactivity: the current concept of the pathophysiology. Low Urin Tract Symptoms. 2014;6(3):131–7.
10. Andersson KE. Current and future drugs for treatment of MS-associated bladder dysfunction. Ann Phys Rehabil Med. 2014;57(5):321–8.
11. Hoag N, Gani J. Underactive bladder: clinical features, urodynamic parameters, and treatment. Int Neurourol J. 2015;19(3):185–9.
12. Kadow BT, Tyagi P, Chermansky CJ. Neurogenic causes of detrusor underactivity. Curr Bladder Dysfunct Rep. 2015;10(4):325–31.
13. Smith PP, Chalmers DJ, Feinn RS. Does defective volume sensation contribute to detrusor underactivity? Neurourol Urodyn. 2015;34(8):752–6.
14. Smith PP, Birder LA, Abrams P, Wein AJ, Chapple CR. Detrusor underactivity and the underactive bladder: symptoms, function, cause-what do we mean? ICI-RS think tank 2014. Neurourol Urodyn. 2016;35(2):312–7.
15. Taylor 3rd JA, Kuchel GA. Detrusor underactivity: clinical features and pathogenesis of an underdiagnosed geriatric condition. J Am Geriatr Soc. 2006;54(12):1920–32.
16. Pfisterer MH, Griffiths DJ, Schaefer W, Resnick NM. The effect of age on lower urinary tract function: a study in women. J Am Geriatr Soc. 2006;54(3):405–12.
17. Collas DM, Malone-Lee JG. Age-associated changes in detrusor sensory function in women with lower urinary tract symptoms. Int Urogynecol J Pelvic Floor Dysfunct. 1996;7(1):24–9.
18. Karram MM, Partoll L, Bilotta V, Angel O. Factors affecting detrusor contraction strength during voiding in women. Obstet Gynecol. 1997;90(5):723–6.
19. Madersbacher S, Pycha A, Schatzl G, Mian C, Klingler CH, Marberger M. The aging lower urinary tract: a comparative urodynamic study of men and women. Urology. 1998;51(2):206–12.
20. Ameda K, Sullivan MP, Bae RJ, Yalla SV. Urodynamic characterization of nonobstructive voiding dysfunction in symptomatic elderly men. J Urol. 1999;162(1):142–6.
21. Malone-Lee J, Wahedna I. Characterisation of detrusor contractile function in relation to old age. Br J Uro. 1993;72(6):873–80.

22. Valentini FA, Robain G, Marti BG. Urodynamics in women from menopause to oldest age: what motive? What diagnosis? Int Braz J Urol. 2011;37(1):100–7.
23. Zimmern P, Litman HJ, Nager CW, Lemack GE, Richter HE, Sirls L, Kraus SR, Sutkin G, Mueller ER. Effect of aging on storage and voiding function in women with stress predominant urinary incontinence. J Urol. 2014;192(2):464–8.
24. Jeong SJ, Kim HJ, Lee YJ, Lee JK, Lee BK, Choo YM, Oh JJ, Lee SC, Jeong CW, Yoon CY, Hong SK, Byun SS, Lee SE. Prevalence and clinical features of detrusor underactivity among elderly with lower urinary tract symptoms: a comparison between men and women. Korean J Urol. 2012;53(5):342–8.
25. Smith PP. Aging and the underactive detrusor: a failure of activity or activation? Neurourol Urodyn. 2010;29(3):408–12.
26. Fry CH, Bayliss M, Young JS, Hussain M. Influence of age and bladder dysfunction on the contractile properties of isolated human detrusor smooth muscle. BJU Int. 2011;108(2 Pt 2):E91–6.
27. Al-Hayek S, Thomas A, Abrams P. Natural history of detrusor contractility--minimum ten-year urodynamic follow-up in men with bladder outlet obstruction and those with detrusor. Scand J Urol Nephrol Suppl. 2004;215:101–8.
28. Abarbanel J, Marcus EL. Impaired detrusor contractility in community-dwelling elderly presenting with lower urinary tract symptoms. Urology. 2007;69(3):436–40.
29. Susset JG, Servot-Viguier D, Lamy F, Madernas P, Black R. Collagen in 155 human bladders. Invest Urol. 1978;16(3):204–6.
30. Elbadawi A. Pathology and pathophysiology of detrusor in incontinence. Urol Clin North Am. 1995;22(3):499–512.
31. Nordling J. The aging bladder--a significant but underestimated role in the development of lower urinary tract symptoms. Exp Gerontol. 2002;37(8–9):991–9.
32. Daneshgari F, Moore C. Diabetic uropathy. Semin Nephrol. 2006;26(2):182–5.
33. Yoshimura N, Chancellor MB, Andersson KE, Christ GJ. Recent advances in understanding the biology of diabetes-associated bladder complications and novel therapy. BJU Int. 2005;95(6):733–8.
34. Daneshgari F, Liu G, Birder L, Hanna-Mitchell AT, Chacko S. Diabetic bladder dysfunction: current translational knowledge. J Urol. 2009;182(6 Suppl):S18–26.
35. Gomez CS, Kanagarajah P, Gousse AE. Bladder dysfunction in patients with diabetes. Curr Urol Rep. 2011;12(6):419–26.
36. Arrellano-Valdez F, Urrutia-Osorio M, Arroyo C, Soto-Vega E. A comprehensive review of urologic complications in patients with diabetes. Springerplus. 2014;3:549.
37. Frimodt-Møller C. Diabetic cystopathy. A review of the urodynamic and clinical features of neurogenic bladder dysfunction in diabetes mellitus. Dan Med Bull. 1978;25(2):49–60.
38. Frimodt-Møller C, Mortensen S. Treatment of diabetic cystopathy. Ann Intern Med. 1980;92(2 Pt 2):327–8.
39. Lifford KL, Curhan GC, Hu FB, Barbieri RL, Grodstein F. Type 2 diabetes mellitus and risk of developing urinary incontinence. J Am Geriatr Soc. 2005;53(11):1851–7.
40. Hill SR, Fayyad AM, Jones GR. Diabetes mellitus and female lower urinary tract symptoms: a review. Neurourol Urodyn. 2008;27:362–7.
41. Sarma AV, Kellogg PJ. Diabetes and benign prostatic hyperplasia: emerging clinical connections. Curr Urol Rep. 2009;10(4):267–75.
42. Sarma AV, St Sauver JL, Hollingsworth JM, Jacobson DJ, McGree ME, Dunn RL, Lieber MM, Jacobsen SJ, Urologic Diseases in America Project. Diabetes treatment and progression of benign prostatic hyperplasia in community-dwelling black and white men. Urology. 2012;79(1):102–8.
43. Fedele D. Therapy insight: sexual and bladder dysfunction associated with diabetes mellitus. Nat Clin Pract Urol. 2005;2(6):282–90.
44. Verrotti A, Prezioso G, Scattoni R, Chiarelli F. Autonomic neuropathy in diabetes mellitus. Front Endocrinol (Lausanne). 2014;5:205.
45. Sasaki K, Chancellor MB, Phelan MW, Yokoyama T, Fraser MO, Seki S, Kubo K, Kumon H, Groat WC, Yoshimura N. Diabetic cystopathy correlates with a long-term decrease in nerve

growth factor levels in the bladder and lumbosacral dorsal root ganglia. J Urol. 2002;168:1259–64.
46. Patel M, Coshall C, Rudd AG, Wolfe CD. Natural history and effects on 2-year outcomes of urinary incontinence after stroke. Stroke. 2001;32(1):122–7.
47. Pizzi A, Falsini C, Martini M, Rossetti MA, Verdesca S, Tosto A. Urinary incontinence after ischemic stroke: clinical and urodynamic studies. Neurourol Urodyn. 2014;33:420.
48. Burney TL, Senapati M, Desai S, Choudhary ST, Badlani GH. Acute cerebrovascular accident and lower urinary tract dysfunction: a prospective correlation of the site of brain injury with urodynamic findings. J Urol. 1996;156:1748–50.
49. Kim TG, Chun MH, Chang MC, Yang S. Outcomes of drug-resistant urinary retention in patients in the early stage of stroke. Ann Rehabil Med. 2015;39:262–7.
50. Kong KH, Young S. Incidence and outcome of post-stroke urinary retention: a prospective study. Arch Phys Med Rehabil. 2000;81:1464–7.
51. Yum KS, Na SJ, Lee KY, Kim J, Oh SH, Kim YD, Yoon B, Heo JH, Lee KO. Pattern of voiding dysfunction after acute brainstem infarction. Eur Neurol. 2013;70:291–6.
52. Cho HJ, Kang TH, Chang JH, Choi YR, Park MG, Choi KD, Sung SM, Park KP, Jung DS. Neuroanatomical correlation of urinary retention in lateral medullary infarction. Ann Neurol. 2015;77:726–33.
53. Ersoz M, Tunc H, Akyuz M, Ozel S. Bladder storage and emptying disorder frequencies in hemorrhagic and ischemic stroke patients with bladder dysfunction. Cerebrovasc Dis. 2005;20:395–9.
54. Yeo L, Singh R, Gundeti M, Barua JM, Masood J. Urinary tract dysfunction in Parkinson's disease: a review. Int Urol Nephrol. 2012;44(2):415–24.
55. Araki I, Kitahara M, Oida T, Kuno S. Voiding dysfunction and Parkinson's disease: urodynamic abnormalities and urinary symptoms. J Urol. 2000;164:1640–16433.
56. Uchiyama T, Sakakibara R, Yamamoto T, Ito T, Yamaguchi C, Awa Y, Yanagisawa M, Higuchi Y, Sato Y, Ichikawa T, Yamanishi T, Hattori T, Kuwabara S. Urinary dysfunction in early and untreated Parkinson's disease. J Neurol Neurosurg Psychiatry. 2011;82(12):1382–6.
57. Liu Z, Uchiyama T, Sakakibara R, Yamamoto T. Underactive and overactive bladders are related to motor function and quality of life in Parkinson's disease. Int Urol Nephrol. 2015;47:751–7.
58. Campeau L, Soler R, Andersson KE. Bladder dysfunction and Parkinsonism: current pathophysiological understanding and management strategies. Curr Urol Rep. 2011;12:396–403.
59. De Ridder D, Van Der Aa F, Debruyne J, D'hooghe MB, Dubois B, Guillaume D, Heerings M, Ilsbroukx S, Medaer R, Nagels G, Seeldrayers P, Van Landegem W, Willekens B, Zicot AF. Consensus guidelines on the neurologist's role in the management of neurogenic lower urinary tract dysfunction in multiple sclerosis. Clin Neurol Neurosurg. 2013;115(10):2033–40.
60. Panicker JN, Fowler CJ. Lower urinary tract dysfunction in patients with multiple sclerosis. Handb Clin Neurol. 2015;130:371–81.
61. Mayo ME, Chetner MP. Lower urinary tract dysfunction in multiple sclerosis. Urology. 1992;39:67–70.
62. Betts CD, D'Mellow MT, Fowler CJ. Urinary symptoms and the neurological features of bladder dysfunction in multiple sclerosis. J Neurol Neurosurg Psychiatry. 1993;56:245–50.
63. Gallien P, Robineau S, Nicolas B, Le Bot MP, Brissot R, Verin M. Vesicourethral dysfunction and urodynamic findings in multiple sclerosis: a study of 149 cases. Arch Phys Med Rehabil. 1998;79:255–7.
64. Litwiller SE, Frohman EM, Zimmern PE. Multiple sclerosis and the urologist. J Urol. 1999;161:743–57.
65. Amarenco G, Raibaut P, Hubeaux K, Jousse M, Sheikh Ismaël S, Lapeyre E. Autonomic nervous system alteration in multiple sclerosis patients with urinary symptoms. Clinical, urodynamic and cardiovascular study. Prog Urol. 2013;23(17):1505–10.
66. Araki I, Matsui M, Ozawa K, Takeda M, Kuno S. Relationship of bladder dysfunction to lesion site in multiple sclerosis. J Urol. 2003;169:1384–7.

67. Ponholzer A, Temml C, Wehrberger C, Marszalek M, Madersbacher S. The association between vascular risk factors and lower urinary tract symptoms in both sexes. Eur Urol. 2006;50:581–6.
68. Yamaguchi O, Nomiya M, Andersson KE. Functional consequences of chronic bladder ischemia. Neurourol Urodyn. 2014;33(1):54–8.
69. Andersson KE, Nomiya M, Yamaguchi O. Chronic pelvic ischemia: contribution to the pathogenesis of lower urinary tract symptoms (LUTS): a New target for pharmacological treatment? Low Urin Tract Symptoms. 2015;7(1):1–8.
70. Camões J, Coelho A, Castro-Diaz D, Cruz F. Lower urinary tract symptoms and aging: the impact of chronic bladder ischemia on overactive bladder syndrome. Urol Int. 2015;95(4):373–9.
71. Thurmond P, Yang JH, Azadzoi KM. Luts in pelvic Ischemia: a new concept in voiding dysfunction. Am J Physiol Renal Physiol. 2016. [Epub ahead of print].
72. Chancellor MB. The overactive bladder progression to underactive bladder hypothesis. Int Urol Nephrol. 2014;46 Suppl 1:S23–7.
73. Nomiya M, Yamaguchi O, Akaihata H, Hata J, Sawada N, Kojima Y, Andersson KE. Progressive vascular damage may lead to bladder underactivity in rats. J Urol. 2014;191:1462–9.
74. Azadzoi KM, Tarcan T, Kozlowski R, Krane RJ, Siroky MB. Overactivity andstructural changes in the chronically ischemic bladder. J Urol. 1999;162:1768–78.
75. Azadzoi KM, Tarcan T, Siroky MB, Krane RJ. Atherosclerosis induced chronic ischemia causes bladder fibrosis and noncompliance in the rabbit. J Urol. 1999;161:1626–35.
76. Nomiya M, Yamaguchi O, Andersson KE, Sagawa K, Aikawa K, Shishido K, Yanagida T, Kushida N, Yazaki J, Takahashi N. The effect of atherosclerosis induced chronic bladder ischemia on bladder function in the rat. Neurourol Urodyn. 2012;31:195–200.
77. Nomiya M, Sagawa K, Yazaki J, Takahashi N, Kushida N, Haga N, Aikawa K, Matsui T, Oka M, Fukui T, Andersson KE, Yamaguchi O. Increased bladder activity is associated with elevated oxidative stress markers and proinflammatory cytokines in a rat model of atherosclerosis-induced chronic bladder ischemia. Neurourol Urodyn. 2012;31:185–9.
78. Azadzoi KM, Shinde VM, Tarcan T, Kozlowski R, Siroky MB. Increased leukotriene and prostaglandin release, and overactivity in the chronically ischemic bladder. J Urol. 2003;169: 1885–91.
79. Azadzoi KM, Yalla SV, Siroky MB. Oxidative stress and neurodegeneration in the ischemic overactive bladder. J Urol. 2007;178:710–5.
80. Nomiya M, Burmeister DM, Sawada N, Campeau L, Zarifpour M, Keys T, Peyton C, Yamaguchi O, Andersson KE. Prophylactic effect of tadalafil on bladder function in a rat model of chronic bladder ischemia. J Urol. 2013;189(2):754–61.
81. Goi Y, Tomiyama Y, Nomiya M, Sagawa K, Aikawa K, Yamaguchi O. Effects of silodosin, a selective α1A-adrenoceptor antagonist, on bladder blood flow and bladder function in a rat model of atherosclerosis induced chronic bladder ischemia without bladder outlet obstruction. J Urol. 2013;190(3):1116–22.
82. Sawada N, Nomiya M, Hood B, Koslov D, Zarifpour M, Andersson KE. Protective effect of a β3-adrenoceptor agonist on bladder function in a rat model of chronic bladder ischemia. Eur Urol. 2013;64(4):664–71.
83. Nomiya M, Burmeister DM, Sawada N, Campeau L, Zarifpour M, Yamaguchi O, Andersson KE. Effect of melatonin on chronic bladder-ischaemia-associated changes in rat bladder function. BJU Int. 2013;112(2):E221–30.

Non-invasive Diagnostics for Detrusor Underactivity/Underactive Bladder

2

Gommert A. van Koeveringe and Kevin L. J. Rademakers

Key Points

- Symptoms and signs cannot accurately make the diagnosis of DU.
- A symptom complex of UAB could potentially capture patients likely to have underlying DU, however the definition is not yet established.
- There is a lack of non invasive diagnostic tests, however penile cuff urodynamics and ultrasonic measurement of detrusor wall thickness show promise, yet require appropriate validation in clinical studies
- In the future, a combined approach that assesses symptoms and signs along with a diagnostic test is likely to be the most practical way forward to the accurate non invasive diagnosis of DU.

Signs of voiding dysfunction such as, elevated post-void residual urine (PVR) and decreased voiding efficiency can be caused by detrusor underactivity (DU), bladder outlet obstruction (BOO) or dysfunctional voiding [1]. These three conditions that may result in voiding dysfunction can up until now only be defined by invasive diagnostic tools using simultaneous measurement of pressure and flow during voiding [1]. During the last three decades, BOO has been the main focus of urodynamic research. Reliable diagnoses of DU, BOO and dysfunctional voiding is currently possible only with formulae or nomograms derived from pressure-flow data [2–5].

G.A. van Koeveringe, MD, PhD (✉)
Professor and Chairman, Department of Urology,
Maastricht University Medical Center+, Maastricht, The Netherlands
e-mail: g.van.koeveringe@mumc.nl

K.L.J. Rademakers
Maastricht University Medical Centre,
Maastricht, The Netherlands
e-mail: kevin.rademakers@mumc.nl

C.R. Chapple et al. (eds.), *Underactive Bladder*,
DOI 10.1007/978-3-319-43087-4_2

Table 2.1 Key symptoms

Symptoms of bladder underactivity	
1	High post void residual
2	Recurrent urinary tract infections
3	Poor or interrupted stream
4	Hesitancy
5	Frequency
6	Urgency

However a urodynamic investigation requires catheter insertion, is bothersome for the patient, time consuming, expensive, and associated with morbidity. In addition urodynamic studies are associated with risks including urinary tract infection, hematuria and urinary retention in up to 19 % of men [6].

Given the disadvantages of standard urodynamics, non-invasive tests and clinical parameters would provide a safer, quicker and cheaper determination of the three types of voiding dysfunctions. However, the diagnosis of the type of voiding dysfunction by analysis of only symptoms and patient characteristics is currently not feasible as LUTS are non-specific for the underlying bladder condition and also age and gender [1, 7, 8]. Clinical parameters such as increased bladder capacity, a palpable bladder or reduced voiding efficiency are indicative for DU but threshold values have not been established yet and bear the risk of also having a lack of specificity by inclusion of patients with BOO and dysfunctional voiding [9, 10].

As DU, and more specifically the contractile capacity of the bladder itself, does not represent all causes of a dysfunction of the bladder, there is a need to define specific index patients and establish differentiating symptoms that may eventually lead to a symptomatic definition. Reduced bladder emptying ability may manifest as both voiding and storage symptoms. Symptoms may include a reduced sensation of bladder fullness, a weak or prolonged stream, hesitancy, interrupted voiding stream, need for straining to start or maintain urinary flow, the feeling of incomplete emptying and recurrent urinary tract infections. Paradoxically, urinary frequency, urgency and incontinence can also occur due to incomplete emptying [9].

The clinical factors should raise the suspicion of underlying DU have been described in a recent review [11] and are presented in Table 2.1.

All symptoms mentioned above are may be related to an DU but can almost equally be attributed to BOO. Therefore, it is a complex task to define a specific complex of symptoms associated with DU. Thus the challenge to accurately define the symptom complex and its context, determine the association of these symptoms to either BOO or DU (or both) and validate such a symptom complex using treatment related outcome measures, is of great importance and has generated much interest.

In an attempt to define a symptom complex analogous to the Overactive bladder, the term Underactive bladder (UAB) has been proposed. A working definition of UAB proposed by a consensus group was "a symptom complex suggestive of the urodynamic diagnosis of detrusor underactivity and characterized by prolonged urination time with or without a sensation of incomplete bladder emptying, usually with hesitancy, reduced sensation on filling and a slow stream[12]. The purpose of the working definition is to clinically detect patients with potential DU [12]. At present both the of the definition UAB and DU are not completely consolidated, however this is still a fast developing field within functional urology. Gammie et al. recently reported the value of symptoms/signs in the identification of DU in a large retrospective series[13]. They showed a significantly higher occurrence of decreased and/or interrupted urinary flow, hesitancy, feeling of incomplete bladder emptying, palpable bladder, and absent and/or decreased sensation in patients with DU compared to patients with normal pressure-flow studies [13]. It remains to be determined whether single symptoms, symptom combinations, or the provisional definition of UAB are useful for the detection of DU in the individual patient [14]. Potential parameters could be high bladder capacity and diminished/absent filling sensation, both of which can be extracted from bladder diaries [12, 13, 15]. In addition, information on bladder capacity and post-void residual is important for the risk assessment of possible consequences of DU. However, to potentially diagnose patients with DU, symptoms seem inadequate and the usage of invasive or other non-invasive additional tools remain necessary.

Recently, studies have been designed to investigate several non-invasive tools for their diagnostic properties in DU. In the past, several of such non-invasive tools have been developed successfully to define BOO/BPO, in which test accuracies between 72 and 88 % were shown [16–18]. Promising, with respect to DU are the usage of penile cuff-urodynamics to measure isovolumetric contraction strength and measurement of detrusor wall thickness [16, 19].

Ultrasound measurement of detrusor wall thickness (DWT) has been shown to be able to diagnose BOO non-invasively [20]. In individuals with BOO, increased DWT is observed in adult men with non-neurogenic LUTS [21–23]. The more severe BOO becomes the greater the DWT [21]. A prospective study demonstrated that a DWT measurement value ≥2 mm in bladders filled ≥250 ml indicates BOO (sensitivity 83 %, specificity 95 %, positive predictive value 94 %, negative predictive value 86 %, likelihood ratio of a positive test result 17.6) [22]. Recently, a pilot study has been performed to assess the possibility of using this technique to identify patients suspected of having DU. This study demonstrated that ultrasound measurement of DWT ≤1.23 mm in combination of bladder capacity >445 ml can detect DU in male patients without BOO or dysfunctional voiding. With these parameters and threshold values this study shows a 100 % association with a DU diagnosis and a confirmation of DU exclusion in 85 % of the patients.

Conclusions

Symptoms and signs alone have not shown specificity for DU. Both BOO and dysfunctional voiding share a similar symptomatology.

Future studies have to determine the clinical importance and threshold values for the diagnosis of DU using non-invasive tests. It is likely that combined use of symptoms and non-invasive tools has to be considered to adequately identify patients with DU.

References

1. Abrams P, Cardozo L, Fall M, et al. The standardisation of terminology of lower urinary tract function: report from the Standardisation Sub-committee of the International Continence Society. Neurourol Urodyn. 2002;21:167–78.
2. van Koeveringe GA, Vahabi B, Andersson KE, et al. Detrusor underactivity: a plea for new approaches to a common bladder dysfunction. Neurourol Urodyn. 2011;30:723–8.
3. Osman NI, Chapple CR, Abrams P, et al. Detrusor underactivity and the underactive bladder: a new clinical entity? A review of current terminology, definitions, epidemiology, aetiology, and diagnosis. Eur Urol. 2013;65:389–98.
4. Oelke M, Rademakers KL, van Koeveringe GA. Detrusor contraction power parameters (BCI and Wmax) rise with increasing bladder outlet obstruction grade in men with lower urinary tract symptoms: results from a urodynamic database analysis. World J Urol. 2014;32:1177–83.
5. Oelke M, Rademakers KL, van Koeveringe GA. Unravelling detrusor underactivity: development of a bladder outlet resistance-bladder contractility nomogram for adult male patients with lower urinary tract symptoms. Neurourol Urodyn. 2015; published online: doi: 10.1002/nau.22841.
6. Klingler HC, Madersbacher S, Djavan B, et al. Morbidity of the evaluation of the lower urinary tract with transurethral multichannel pressure-flow studies. J Urol. 1998;159:191–4.
7. el Din KE, Kiemeney LA, de Wildt MJ, et al. The correlation between bladder outlet obstruction and lower urinary tract symptoms as measured by the international prostate symptom score. J Urol. 1996;156:1020–5.
8. Schäfer W, Rübben H, Noppeney R, Deutz FJ. Obstructed and unobstructed prostatic obstruction. A plea for urodynamic objectivation for bladder outflow obstruction in benign prostatic hyperplasia. World J Urol. 1989;6:198–203.
9. Taylor JA, Kuchel GA. Detrusor underactivity: clinical features and pathogenesis of an underdiagnosed geriatric condition. J Am Geriatr Soc. 2006;54:1920–32.
10. Gammie A, Kaper M, Dorrepaal C, et al. Signs and symptoms of detrusor underactivity: an analysis of clinical presentation and urodynamic tests from a large group of patients undergoing pressure flow studies. Eur Urol. 2016;69(2):361–9. doi:10.1016/j.eururo.2015.08.014. published online.
11. van Koeveringe GA, Rademakers KL. Factors impacting bladder underactivity and clinical implications. Minerva Urol Nefrol. 2015;67(2):139–48.
12. Chapple CR, et al. The underactive bladder: a New clinical concept? Eur Urol. 2015;68(3):351–3.
13. Smith PP. Aging and the underactive detrusor: a failure of activity or activation? Neurourol Urodyn. 2010;29(3):408–12.
14. Rademakers K, van Koeveringe G, Oelke M. Symptomatic differences in non-obstructive patients with poor detrusor function versus normal detrusor function. In International Continence Society annual meeting, Montreal, 2015.
15. Smith PP, Chalmers DJ, Feinn RS. Does defective volume sensation contribute to detrusor underactivity? Neurourol Urodyn. 2015;34(8):752–6.
16. McIntosh SL, et al. Noninvasive assessment of bladder contractility in men. J Urol. 2004;172 (4 Pt 1):1394–8.
17. Kessler TM, et al. Ultrasound assessment of detrusor thickness in men-can it predict bladder outlet obstruction and replace pressure flow study? J Urol. 2006;175(6):2170–3.
18. De Nunzio C, et al. The diagnosis of benign prostatic obstruction: validation of the young academic urologist clinical nomogram. Urology. 2015;86(5):1032–6.
19. Oelke M, R.K, van Koeveringe G. Non-invasive clinical indicators of detrusor underactivity in adult men – results of a pilot study. J Urol. 2014; 191 Suppl :E887.
20. Belal M, Abrams P. Noninvasive methods of diagnosing bladder outlet obstruction in men. Part 1: nonurodynamic approach. J Urol. 2006;176:22–8.
21. Oelke M, Höfner K, Wiese B, et al. Increase in detrusor wall thickness indicates bladder outlet obstruction (BOO) in men. World J Urol. 2002;19:443–52.
22. Oelke M, Höfner K, Jonas U, et al. Diagnostic accuracy of noninvasive tests to evaluate bladder outlet obstruction in men: detrusor wall thickness, uroflowmetry, postvoid residual urine, and prostate volume. Eur Urol. 2007;52:827–34.
23. Arnolds M, Oelke M. Positioning invasive versus noninvasive urodynamics in the assessment of bladder outlet obstruction. Curr Opin Urol. 2009;19:55–62.

3 Invasive Diagnostic Tests

Altaf Mangera

Key Points

- Invasive pressure flow urodynamics are the only available method to diagnose DU
- Several measures to assess detrusor contraction strength are available, including mathematical calculation, indices and urodynamic stop-tests. All rely on the bladder outlet relation, the inverse relationship between pressure and flow.
- Other aspects of bladder contraction may also be important including the speed and duration of contraction however these aspects are even less well characterised than contraction strength.
- Ambulatory urodynamics can be helpful in differentiating those with "bashful bladder" from patients with true DU.

Introduction

The bladder is considered an "unreliable witness" and the only accepted modality for clinically estimating bladder function is an invasive urodynamic study. However, there are currently no universally agreed criteria for diagnosing DUA. In this section, we discuss the parameters described in diagnosing DUA.

A. Mangera, FRCS(Urol), MD, FEBU
Department of Urology, Sheffield Teaching Hospitals, Sheffield, UK
e-mail: mangeraaltaf@hotmail.com

C.R. Chapple et al. (eds.), *Underactive Bladder*,
DOI 10.1007/978-3-319-43087-4_3

Detrusor Contraction Strength

Most data regarding the diagnosis of DUA is based on assessing detrusor contraction strength. However, the detrusor contraction generates both pressure and flow and so both parameters Pdet@Qmax and Qmax are used to diagnose DUA [1]. Both need to be reduced below the "normal" ranges for the particular patient group for DUA. For men, the ranges were extrapolated from those who underwent bladder outflow obstruction surgery [2, 3]. In healthy men and women these ranges are less well characterized [4–6].

Besides the fact that it only represents a specific group of men, there are other limitations with this approach. Firstly, it only takes account of one point in the voiding cycle. Voiding is a dynamic process and the reading of two parameters at exactly one time point excludes the majority of the void. Secondly, it is likely to underestimate the contraction strength due to the bladder outlet relation (BOR); the normal inverse relationship between detrusor pressure and urine flow [7]. Based on the Hill equation, the BOR principle states that for an actively contracting muscle during voiding- when the flow is low the pressure is high and vice versa. On this principle the pdet@Qmax actually represents the point of least pressure. Thirdly, the variability in bladder outlet resistance which affects flow rate is not considered as bladder outlet resistance is not measured. Thus a low Qmax due to reduced outlet resistance (e.g. post-prostatectomy incontinence) may result in a normal Qmax.

Therefore, to more accurately assess detrusor contraction strength methods were developed to estimate isovolumetric pressure. These are based on mechanical or volitional interruption to the urinary stream during an urodynamic study [8]. Alternatively post hoc mathematical calculations may be used to infer the isovolumetric pressure. Many of these are of limited use in clinical practice due to their complexity and impracticality.

The Watts factor = $[(pdet + a)\ (vdet + b) - ab]/2\pi]$ is an estimate of the power per unit area of bladder surface that is generated by the detrusor, corrected for the finite power required for either isometric contraction or for shortening against no load. Derived from experimental data, vdet is detrusor shortening velocity and a and b are fixed constants (a = 25 cmH_2O, b = 6 mm/s) [9]. Throughout the voiding cycle the WF varies due to the variation in pdet and vdet. The point proposed to best represent detrusor contraction strength is the maximal WF. The major advantages of the WF are that it is not affected by increased outlet resistance[10] and also it minimally depends on volume [9]. However, currently no cut offs are validated for the normal and abnormal ranges, but based on expert opinion- 7 W/m^2 and above has been suggested [11]. A study of 786 men with varying degrees of BOO showed that the WF continuously increased with the grade of BOO [12]. Therefore, it was suggested that a single threshold value was inappropriate and the degree of BOO would need to be factored in. The WF, however is not in everyday clinical use due to the complexity of the calculation. The other major limitation is that it does not consider how well sustained a contraction is.

Extrapolating on the BOR principle, Schäfer superimposed his pressure flow nomogram which estimates the isometric contraction strength. The BOR is simplified and read off the Y-axis (which represents the isometric pressure- pdet) by projecting a parallel line back from the point representing pdet Qmax. This projected isovolumetric pressure (PIP) can be calculated by the following formula $PIP = Pdet@$

Qmax + KQmax, where is K a fixed constant representing the slope of the BOR[13]. The value of K is dependent on the specific population studied, in men with BPH it is taken as 5 cmH_2O/ml/s whilst in older women 1 cmH_2O/ml/s was found to be more accurate[8]. Based on this the suggested formula for use in men in clinical practice is: *PIP = Pdet@Qmax + 5Qmax* and in older women *Pdet@Qmax + Qmax*. In men, A PIP of >150 represents strong contractility, 100–150 normal contractility, 50–100 weak contractility and <50 very weak contractility. The corresponding BOR's at these cut offs were plotted on the Schäfer's pressure flow nomogram, to give subdivisions for contractility.

Subsequently, Abrams described the bladder contractility index (BCI), which uses the same formula as PIP and is instead divided into three groups (strong >150, normal 100–150 and weak <100) [14]. Evidently all these methods are fairly easy and quick to calculate, but tend to overestimate PIP, as adjustments need to be made for use in different populations. Although test-retest reliability is thought to be acceptable it is less consistent than measures that directly record isovolumetric pressures [15].

Isovolumetric pressure may be measured directly by mechanically obstructing urine flow [16]. This can be achieved either through (1) a stop test, stoppage of urine flow after it has begun, or (2) a continuous occlusion test, where the urine outflow is blocked before and during the course of the voiding contraction.

A voluntary stop test requires a patient to voluntarily contract the urethral sphincter after commencement of voiding, whereas in a mechanical stop test the bladder outflow is occluded by the investigator (e.g. by tugging a catheter balloon against the bladder neck). Both these techniques correlate well with each other in both genders [15] but the voluntary stop test tends to produce a lower value for isovolumetric pressure by approximately 20 cmH_2O. This is probably explained by the reflex detrusor inhibition induced by voluntary urethral sphincter contraction [17]. The voluntary stop test is difficult and sometimes impossible to conduct in patients with urethral sphincter weakness.

The continuous occlusion test has greater test retest reliability and allows assessment of contraction sustainability. The limitation is that you do not obtain a representative flow measurement during that particular contraction. Although it correlates well with the ability to empty the bladder [18], continuous occlusion is potentially painful and has found little acceptance outside of a research setting.

Detrusor Contraction Speed

A bladder that contracts more slowly could, in theory, result in clinical symptoms which presumably would lead to an increase in voiding time, although this is considered not part of the ICS definition. A reduction in detrusor shortening velocity (calculated by the formula $vdet = Q/2[3/(V + Vt)/4\pi]^{0.66}$ where Q represents the flow rate (ml/s), V represents bladder volume (ml) and Vt represents the volume of non-contracting bladder wall tissue) was found to precede reduction in Watt factor in series of longitudinal studies in both males [19, 20] and females [21]. The utility of calculating detrusor contraction speed in diagnosing DUA is however limited.

Detrusor Contraction Duration/Bladder Sensation

A detrusor contraction of reduced duration is suggested by the ICS as part of the definition of DUA [22], however the limits of a normal voiding detrusor contraction are not defined. There are only a few studies that assess the duration of contraction as a urodynamic parameter. In a study of men with BPH, unobstructed patients with poor contractility actually had significantly longer contraction durations than those with no obstruction and normal contractility [23].

It is likely that the contraction duration reflects the underlying pathophysiological mechanisms, for example, an early termination of the micturition reflex could presumably lead to a shorter duration. It is thought that loss of afferent sensation from the bladder reaching the brain due to interruption at either bladder, spinal cord or higher levels prevents the bladder from being emptied completely due to loss of stretch/proprioceptive input. This is likely to manifest as high/variable residual volumes. Also an interrupted detrusor contraction pattern may occur if the sphincter contracts concomitantly and thus switches off the voiding reflex and in some patients it may be switched off altogether.

As the afferent nerves play such a central role in the initiation and maintenance of a detrusor contraction it is worth discussing how they can be assessed urodynamically. Traditionally, the urodynamicist assesses the patient's perceptions of bladder filling e.g. first sensation, first desire, strong desire and capacity. Thresholds in normal individuals are available [24], although this method can be criticized as patients may report bladder sensation even when the bladder is not being filled [25, 26] and as with any subjective measure, there is substantial individual variation, due the false circumstances of the study and the anxiety of the subject.

Sensory responses to the passage of electrical current through the bladder wall (current perception threshold testing) may provide a more objective measure but is clearly rather an invasive approach and is as yet an unvalidated research technique. Also it does not assess the sensations of filling as such and may not be so relevant. Moreover, a standardized method for measuring the duration of the detrusor contraction and bladder sensations along with normal cut offs is required before any conclusions can be reached.

Ambulatory Urodynamics

Patients often fail to void during an urodynamic study due to anxiety or a so called "bashful bladder". It is thought this arises due to poor pelvic floor relaxation and reflex detrusor inhibition. Alternatively the patient may have true DUA or acontractile detrusor. A careful history is usually sufficient to differentiate between the two situations. Where there is doubt ambulatory urodynamics may be useful [27]. Van Koevering et al. demonstrated 84 % of patients who failed to generate a detrusor contraction during standard urodynamics had evidence of demonstrable contraction during an ambulatory study [28]. Therefore ambulatory urodynamics clearly has a role in this patient cohort.

Summary

Assessing detrusor contraction strength at one point (pdet@Qmax) in relation to the Qmax has gained most popularity due to standardization by the ICS. This however, as discussed above, has its limitations. Although it is simple and largely reproducible not all patients will fit neatly into the defined categories.

It is certain that DUA is due to a number of pathophysiological mechanisms and cannot be thought of alone without considering the sphincter mechanism and afferent sensation. It is important to remember to take a good history from the patient and form a set of questions which the urodynamics may be able to objectively test against standardized sets of the population.

Besides detrusor contraction strength, detrusor contraction duration is also likely to play a role in how well a bladder empties. Currently we are lacking standardized data of detrusor contraction duration and an equation involving contraction strength with duration may be a way forward.

We have summarized the current methods of assessing DUA in the table below.

Type	Method	Advantages	Disadvantages
Mathematical calculations	Watts factor	1. Measure of bladder power 2. Minimally dependant on volume of urine	1. Lengthy and complex calculation 2. No validated thresholds 3. Does not measure sustainability of contraction 4. Affected by BOO
	Detrusor shortening velocity	1. May identify early stage DU	
Indices	Detrusor contraction Coefficient (DECO)	1. Simple to use 2. measurement easy to obtain 3. estimation of isolumetric contraction	1. Does not measure sustainability of contraction 2. May not be applicable to other groups
	Bladder contractility index (BCI)		
Occlusion testing	Voluntary stop test	1. Real time indication of isovolumetric contraction strength 2. no calculations	1. Uncomfortable or painful for patients 2. Impractical 3. No information on sustainability of contraction in (in continuous occlusion) 4. May underestimate isovolumetric pressure (stop test) 5. Unusable in some patient groups
	Mechanical stop test		
	Continuous occlusion		
Ranges of urodynamic measurements	Pdet@Qmax (e.g.<40) Qmax (e.g.<15)	1. Simple to use	1. No widely accepted "normal" ranges 2. Underestimate contraction strength 3. Does not conceptually consider co-existence of BOO and DU

Reproduced from Osman et al. [29], with permission

References

1. Griffiths DJ. Editorial: bladder failure–a condition to reckon with. J Urol. 2003;169(3):1011–2.
2. Abrams PH, Griffiths DJ. The assessment of prostatic obstruction from urodynamic measurements and from residual urine. Br J Urol. 1979;51(2):129–34.
3. Schafer W, Waterbär F, Langen PH, et al. A simplified graphic procedure for detailed analysis of detrusor and outlet function during voiding. Neurourol Urodyn. 1989;8:405–7.
4. Rosario DJ, Woo HH, Chapple CR. Definition of normality of pressure-flow parameters based on observations in asymptomatic men. Neurourol Urodyn. 2008;27(5):388–94.
5. Schmidt F, et al. Urodynamic patterns of normal male micturition: influence of water consumption on urine production and detrusor function. J Urol. 2002;168(4 Pt 1):1458–63.
6. Pfisterer MH, et al. The effect of age on lower urinary tract function: a study in women. J Am Geriatr Soc. 2006;54(3):405–12.
7. Griffiths DJ. The mechanics of the urethra and of micturition. Br J Urol. 1973;45(5):497–507.
8. Griffiths D. Detrusor contractility--order out of chaos. Scand J Urol Nephrol Suppl. 2004;215:93–100.
9. DJ G. Assesment of detrusor contraction strenght or contractility. Neurourol Urodyn. 1991;10:1–18.
10. Lecamwasam HS, et al. The maximum watts factor as a measure of detrusor contractility independent of outlet resistance. Neurourol Urodyn. 1998;17(6):621–35.
11. van Koeveringe GA, et al. Detrusor underactivity: a plea for new approaches to a common bladder dysfunction. Neurourol Urodyn. 2011;30(5):723–8.
12. Oelke M, Rademakers KL, van Koeveringe GA. Detrusor contraction power parameters (BCI and W max) rise with increasing bladder outlet obstruction grade in men with lower urinary tract symptoms: results from a urodynamic database analysis. World J Urol. 2014;32(5):1177–83.
13. Schafer W. Analysis of bladder-outlet function with the linearized passive urethral resistance relation, linPURR, and a disease-specific approach for grading obstruction: from complex to simple. World J Urol. 1995;13(1):47–58.
14. Abrams P. Bladder outlet obstruction index, bladder contractility index and bladder voiding efficiency: three simple indices to define bladder voiding function. BJU Int. 1999;84(1):14–5.
15. Tan TL, et al. Which stop test is best? Measuring detrusor contractility in older females. J Urol. 2003;169(3):1023–7.
16. Sullivan M, Yalla SV. Functional studies to assess bladder contractility. J urol Urogynakol. 2007;14(1):7–10.
17. Sullivan MP, et al. Continuous occlusion test to determine detrusor contractile performance. J Urol. 1995;154(5):1834–40.
18. Sullivan MP, Yalla SV. Detrusor contractility and compliance characteristics in adult male patients with obstructive and nonobstructive voiding dysfunction. J Urol. 1996;155(6):1995–2000.
19. Cucchi A, et al. Urodynamic findings suggesting two-stage development of idiopathic detrusor underactivity in adult men. Urology. 2007;70(1):75–9.
20. Cucchi A, Quaglini S, Rovereto B. Different evolution of voiding function in underactive bladders with and without detrusor overactivity. J Urol. 2010;183(1):229–33.
21. Cucchi A, Quaglini S, Rovereto B. Development of idiopathic detrusor underactivity in women: from isolated decrease in contraction velocity to obvious impairment of voiding function. Urology. 2008;71(5):844–8.
22. Abrams P, et al. The standardisation of terminology of lower urinary tract function: report from the Standardisation Sub-committee of the International Continence Society. Neurourol Urodyn. 2002;21(2):167–78.
23. Ameda K, et al. Detrusor contraction duration as a urodynamic parameter of bladder outlet obstruction for evaluating men with lower urinary tract symptoms. J Urol. 1998;160(2):482–6.

24. Wyndaele JJ. The normal pattern of perception of bladder filling during cystometry studied in 38 young healthy volunteers. J Urol. 1998;160(2):479–81.
25. Erdem E, et al. How reliable are bladder perceptions during cystometry? Neurourol Urodyn. 2004;23(4):306–9; discussion 10.
26. De Wachter S, Van Meel TD, Wyndaele JJ. Can a faked cystometry deceive patients in their perception of filling sensations? A study on the reliability of spontaneously reported cystometric filling sensations in patients with non-neurogenic lower urinary tract dysfunction. Neurourol Urodyn. 2008;27(5):395–8.
27. Rosario DJ, et al. Urodynamic assessment of the bashful bladder. J Urol. 2000;163(1):215–20.
28. van Koeveringe GA, Rahnama'i MS, Berghmans BC. The additional value of ambulatory urodynamic measurements compared with conventional urodynamic measurements. BJU Int. 2010;105(4):508–13.
29. Osman NI, Chapple CR, Abrams P, et al. Detrusor underactivity and the underactive bladder: a new clinical entity? A review of current terminology, definitions, epidemiology, aetiology, and diagnosis. Eur Urol. 2014;65(2):389–98.

Epidemiology of Underactive Bladder

4

Nadir I. Osman, Christopher J. Hillary,
and Christopher R. Chapple

Key Points

- DU and BOO overlap considerably in terms of symptoms and signs which makes it difficult to understand their relative contributions to symptoms on a population perspective.
- DU commonly occurs with other urodynamic diagnoses such BOO and stress urinary incontinence.
- DU is common in both men and women presenting with LUTS and increases in prevalence with ageing.
- The limited available evidence suggest that DU is not necessarily a progressive problem in men, although studies looking at the natural history are lacking.

Introduction

Many epidemiological studies have established that lower urinary tract symptoms (LUTS) are a highly significant health problem across the world. LUTS show an increase in prevalence with ageing and are commonly categorized as voiding, storage or post micturition. In population-based studies, storage symptoms are often related to the Detrusor overactivity (DO) and the overactive bladder (OAB) symptom complex whilst voiding LUTS are often attributed to bladder outlet obstruction (BOO) secondary to benign prostatic enlargement (BPE) for which prevalence evidence is available from clinical and pathological studies. As yet no epidemiological

N.I. Osman (✉) • C.J. Hillary • C.R. Chapple
Department of Urology, Royal Hallamshire Hospital, Glossop Road, Sheffield, UK
e-mail: nadirosman@hotmail.com; c.hillary@sheffield.ac.uk; c.r.chapple@shef.ac.uk

C.R. Chapple et al. (eds.), *Underactive Bladder*,
DOI 10.1007/978-3-319-43087-4_4

studies have assessed the contribution of detrusor underactivity (DU) to the occurrence of LUTS. The primary reason for this is that DU is a diagnosis that requires an invasive pressure flow urodynamic study, hence it has been unfeasible to collect population data due to the obvious impracticalities of performing such studies in large groups of people, the majority of whom are asymptomatic. The result of this has been our very limited understanding of the incidence, prevalence, aetiological factors and natural history of DU.

Challenges in Acquiring Epidemiological Data

Due to the impracticality of performing urodynamic studies on a population basis it is worthwhile looking at non-invasive potential proxy measures. As noted above, most epidemiological studies are based on symptoms, however the symptoms that we commonly associate with DU such as reduced urinary flow, straining and hesitancy are all prevalent with patients with BOO. Even patients with the OAB may experience these voiding symptoms due to urinary frequency resulting in reduced voided volumes. Nevertheless in a recent cross sectional survey of 633 men and women age 33–92 years old in the United States, 23 % of respondents reported difficulty emptying their bladder suggesting that symptoms associated DU are common in the general population [1].

Uroflowmetry is a potential non invasive marker but using current methods cannot reliably distinguish DU from BOO [2] or attest to the relative contribution of either in cases where both dysfunctions are present. Similarly a raised post voiding residual as commonly measured using an ultrasound scan cannot differentiate between DU and BOO [3].

Urinary retention is a common urological diagnosis for which at face value it would be relatively easy to collect population data using hospital based diagnostic coding.

However urinary retention remains a rather nebulous concept, which is commonly categorized into acute or chronic and attributed to BOO, DU or a combination. Chronic retention is concept that is commonly related to DU, historically defined as a PVR over 300 ml. The International Continence Society (ICS) does not specifiy a threshold volume in their most recent standardization report, defining it as "a non painful bladder, which remains palpable or percussable after the patient has passed urine"[4]. In common with the other potential non invasive markers of DU, it is not possible to certain the relative contributions of DU and BOO. In summary there is currently no reliable non invasive method of establishing the epidemiology of DU.

The Relationship Between DU and BOO

In male LUTS the overwhelming focus of research has been on the BPE leading to BOO hypothesis as the cause of symptoms and urinary retention despite the common perception that a significant minority, an estimated at 10–20 %, of men with impaired flow on presentation have at least a degree of DU [5]. At present we do not entirely understand the relationship between BOO and DU, while it is clear that not all men with BOO develop DU, not all men with DU have concomitant BOO [6]. Certainly, it has long been held that DU results as a consequence of prolonged BOO which gives rise to structural and functional bladder wall changes leading to loss of normal bladder contractility as demonstrated in many small mammal studies. In some patients DU may represent an entirely independent disease process, such as a sensory problem, as has been theorized to occur in men with chronic retention who remain relatively symptom free until a late stage [7].

Although in male LUTS it is challenging to assess the relative contribution of BOO and DU on a population perspective, in women BOO is far less common due to the absence of a prostate gland and is estimated to occur in only 2.7 % of those referred to secondary care with LUTS [8]. The implication of this is that voiding symptoms or retention in women is more likely to be due to DU. The aetiology of BOO in women most commonly comprised of post-incontinence surgery BOO, urethral stricture, pelvic organ prolapse, urethral diverticule and gynaecological pelvic masses

The Relationship Between DU and DO/OAB

Due to the common occurrence of DU and DO and the association of both with ageing, BOO and Diabetes Mellitus it is possible the two diagnosis are linked. It is certainly the case that the two diagnoses can occur simultaneously, particularly in the institutionalised elderly in the form Detrusor hyperactivity impaired contractility (DHIC) as described by Resnick and Yalla [9]. Some have suggested that DO to DU progression may occur as result of bladder wall and sensory nerve changes, although this is largely hypothetical with no convincing evidence [10].

Prevalence of DU in Clinical Studies

In the absence of any reliable epidemiological studies, prevalence data can be derived from studies where urodynamic studies are performed in patients presenting with LUTS. Several such studies are available for review and are outlined in Table 4.1. Summarizing this data it is apparent than in patients with non-neurogenic LUTS undergoing pressure flow urodynamics DU, variably defined, is present in 9–28 % of men younger than 50 year increasing to 48 % in men older than 70 year. In elderly women, the prevalence ranges from 12 to 45 %, peaking in those in care and nursing homes where the entity of Detrusor hyperactivity impaired contractility (DHIC) is an important cause of incontinence.

Such retrospective analysis of series of patients have limitations as they often rely upon post-hoc interpretation of urodynamic traces [24] which along with the variability in definitions used makes application to the general population not possible. Nevertheless the findings do suggest that DU occurs with sufficient frequency to be seriously considered as a possible cause of LUTS in patients.

Table 4.1 Prevalence of detrusor underactivity in clinical studies

Study	Population	Size	Age range (yrs)	Diagnostic criteria	Prevalence of DU + (% of acontractile detrusors)
Fusco et al. (2001) [11]	Male	541	26–89	pdet@Qmax ≤30 and Qmax ≤12	10 %
Kuo et al. (2007) [12]	Male	1407	46–96	Relaxed sphincter EMG with open membranous urethra during voiding and low flow rate	10.6 %
Nitti et al. (2002) [13]	Male	85	18–45	Bladder outlet obstruction index <20 and uroflow <12 ml/s	9 %
Wang et al. (2003) [14]	Male	90	18–50	pdet@Qmax <30, Qmax <15	10 %
Kaplan et al. (1996) [15]	Male	137	18–50	pdet@Qmax <45 cm and Qmax < 12 ml	23 % (5 %)
Karami et al. (2011) [16]	Male	456	18–40	ICS definition	12.9 % (10.5 %)
Arbabanel et al. (2007) [17]	Male Female	82 99	>70 >70	Pdet@Qmax < 30cmH_2O and Qmax < 10 ml	48 % 12 %
Jeong et al. (2012) [18]	Male Female	632 547	>65 >65	Bladder contractility index <100 (men) Qmax ≤ 12, Pdet@Qmax ≤ 10 (women)	40.2 % 13.3 %
Resnick et al. (1989) [19]	Male Female (Institutionalized)	17 77	87	In the absence of obstruction, Underactive detrusor: “Failure to empty in the absence of an increase abdominal pressure”. DHIC: “Involuntary detrusor contraction that emptied less than half of volume instilled”	41.2 % 37.7 %
Resnick et al. (1996) [20]	Female (institutionalized)	97	87.6[b]	“Reproducible failure of the involuntary contraction to empty at least half of bladder contents in the absence of straining, urethral obstruction, and detrusor-sphincter dyssynergia”	45 %[b]
Groutz et al. (1999) [21]	Female	206	62.6 ± 15.8 years[a]	ICS definition	19 %
Valentini et al. (2011) [22]	Female	442	>55	“impaired detrusor contraction leading to prolonged voiding time and high residual volume”	13.8 %

Reproduced from Osman et al. [23], with permission

[a]Mean ± SD

[b]DHIC

Jeong and colleagues reported one of the biggest clinical urodynamic series studying 1,179 men and women over the age of 65 years [18]. The results showed that DU defined as bladder contractility index <100 in men and Qmax ≤12, Pdet@Qmax ≤10 in women, frequently occurs along with other urodynamic diagnoses in older individuals Of men, 46.5 % with DU also had DOA or BOO whilst in women 72.6 % of those with DU also had DOA or urodynamic stress urinary incontinence.

The Natural History of DU

There is sparse data available to establish the natural history of DU. One such study was performed by the group in Bristol (UK), who reported a over decade long follow up of adult males who were originally diagnosed with DU using the urodynamic criteria Qmax <15 ml/s and Pdet@Qmax <40cmH_2O [6]. These patients were all managed with an initial conservative watchful waiting approach and not operated on or catheterized. The findings showed that overall in the 69 men studied no significant worsening in symptoms or urodynamic findings occurred. Eleven men decided to go undergo transurethral resection of the prostate, 8 (11.6 %) due to worsening LUTS and 3 (4.35 %) due to acute urinary retention. In those with worsening LUTS the repeat urodynamic studies before operation showed no change from baseline parameters.

From this study we can surmise that DU is not necessarily a progressive phenomenon in most men with no neurological disease. It is interesting to note that the mean PVR at the end of 10 years follow up in this group was 108–126 ml suggesting that DU may not necessarily lead to Chronic retention as commonly defined. This suggests DU and chronic retention may have separate underlying aetiological factors. Further studies are clearly needed to establish the natural history of DU in different groups.

Conclusions

Very little is known of the epidemiology of DU. The overlap with symptoms and signs of BOO has hampered the ability to acquire good quality epidemiological data. Developing a more robust definition of underactive bladder (UAB) as a the symptom complex associated with DU may in future facilitate population studies allowing us to achieve a better understanding of the risk factors, associations and natural history of the condition. However for the time being clinical urodynamic series have shown us that DU is very common in the group of patients referred for urodynamic studies to warrant serious consideration as cause of symptoms in both men and women.

References

1. Valente S, DuBeau C, Chancellor D, Okonski J, Vereecke A, Doo F, et al. Epidemiology and demographics of the underactive bladder: a cross-sectional survey. Int Urol Nephrol. 2014;46 Suppl 1:S7–10.
2. Chancellor MB, Blaivas JG, Kaplan SA, Axelrod S. Bladder outlet obstruction versus impaired detrusor contractility: the role of outflow. J Urol. 1991;145:810–2.

3. Abrams PH, Griffiths DJ. The assessment of prostatic obstruction from urodynamic measurements and from residual urine. Br J Urol. 1979;51:129–34.
4. Abrams P, Cardozo L, Fall M, Griffiths D, Rosier P, Ulmsten U, et al. The standardisation of terminology of lower urinary tract function: report from the Standardisation Sub-committee of the International Continence Society. Neurourol Urodyn. 2002;21:167–78.
5. Abrams P. Urodynamics. 3rd ed. London: Springer; 2006.
6. Thomas AW, Cannon A, Bartlett E, Ellis-Jones J, Abrams P. The natural history of lower urinary tract dysfunction in men: minimum 10-year urodynamic follow-up of untreated detrusor underactivity. BJU Int. 2005;96:1295–300.
7. Parys BT, Machin DG, Woolfenden KA, Parsons KF. Chronic urinary retention–a sensory problem? Br J Urol. 1988;62:546–9.
8. Massey JA, Abrams PH. Obstructed voiding in the female. Br J Urol. 1988;61:36–9.
9. Resnick NM, Yalla SV. Detrusor hyperactivity with impaired contractile function. An unrecognized but common cause of incontinence in elderly patients. JAMA. 1987;257:3076–81.
10. Chancellor MB. The overactive bladder progression to underactive bladder hypothesis. Int Urol Nephrol. 2014;46 Suppl 1:S23–7.
11. Fusco F, Groutz A, Blaivas JG, Chaikin DC, Weiss JP. Videourodynamic studies in men with lower urinary tract symptoms: a comparison of community based versus referral urological practices. J Urol. 2001;166:910–3.
12. Kuo HC. Videourodynamic analysis of pathophysiology of men with both storage and voiding lower urinary tract symptoms. Urology. 2007;70:272–6.
13. Nitti VW, Lefkowitz G, Ficazzola M, Dixon CM. Lower urinary tract symptoms in young men: videourodynamic findings and correlation with noninvasive measures. J Urol. 2002;168:135–8.
14. Wang CC, Yang SS, Chen YT, Hsieh JH. Videourodynamics identifies the causes of young men with lower urinary tract symptoms and low uroflow. Eur Urol. 2003;43:386–90.
15. Kaplan SA, Ikeguchi EF, Santarosa RP, D'Alisera PM, Hendricks J, Te AE, et al. Etiology of voiding dysfunction in men less than 50 years of age. Urology. 1996;47:836–9.
16. Karami H, Valipour R, Lotfi B, Mokhtarpour H, Razi A. Urodynamic findings in young men with chronic lower urinary tract symptoms. NeurourolUrodyn. 2011;30:1580–5.
17. Abarbanel J, Marcus EL. Impaired detrusor contractility in community-dwelling elderly presenting with lower urinary tract symptoms. Urology. 2007;69:436–40.
18. Jeong SJ, Kim HJ, Lee YJ, Lee JK, Lee BK, Choo YM, et al. Prevalence and clinical features of detrusor underactivity among elderly with lower urinary tract symptoms: a comparison between Men and women. Korean J Urol. 2012;53:342–8.
19. Resnick NM, Yalla SV, Laurino E. The pathophysiology of urinary incontinence among institutionalized elderly persons. N Engl J Med. 1989;320:1–7.
20. Resnick NM, Brandeis GH, Baumann MM, DuBeau CE, Yalla SV. Misdiagnosis of urinary incontinence in nursing home women: prevalence and a proposed solution. NeurourolUrodyn. 1996;15:599–613. discussion –8.
21. Groutz A, Gordon D, Lessing JB, Wolman I, Jaffa A, David MP. Prevalence and characteristics of voiding difficulties in women: are subjective symptoms substantiated by objective urodynamic data? Urology. 1999;54:268–72.
22. Valentini FA, Robain G, Marti BG. Urodynamics in women from menopause to oldest age: what motive? What diagnosis? Int Braz J Urol Off J Braz Soc Urol. 2011;37:100–7.
23. Osman NI, Chapple CR, Abrams P, et al. Detrusor underactivity and the underactive bladder: a new clinical entity? A review of current terminology definitions, epidemiology, aetiology, and diagnosis. Eur Urol. 2014;65(2):389–98.
24. Smith PP, Hurtado EA, Appell RA. Post hoc interpretation of urodynamic evaluation is qualitatively different than interpretation at the time of urodynamic study. NeurourolUrodyn. 2009;28:998–1002.

5 Indications for Treatment

Christopher J. Hillary, Nadir I. Osman, and Christopher R. Chapple

Key Points

- Patients with DU fit in two clinically relevant categories: those with symptoms but not reliant on catheterisation to achieve bladder emptying and those who rely on catheterisation (intermittent or indwelling for bladder emptying).
- Indications for treatment in patients with DU include bothersome symptoms, incomplete bladder emptying resulting in urinary retention, recurrent urinary tract infection or renal impairment.
- There is no available validated patient reported outcome measure with which to assess patients with DU undergoing surgery.
- Factors associate with poor outcomes following surgery include older age (>80), high post void residual (>1500 ml) and low voiding pressure.
- Men with DU undergoing surgical therapy require thorough pre-operative counselling as the outcomes are poorer than in men with preserved bladder contractility.

C.J. Hillary • N.I. Osman (✉) • C.R. Chapple
Department of Urology, The Royal Hallamshire Hospital, Sheffield, UK
e-mail: c.hillary@sheffield.ac.uk; nadirosman@hotmail.com; c.r.chapple@shef.ac.uk

C.R. Chapple et al. (eds.), *Underactive Bladder*,
DOI 10.1007/978-3-319-43087-4_5

Introduction

Owing to the plethora of symptoms with which patients with detrusor underactivity (DU) can suffer and the current lack of a DU-specific validated patient reported outcome measure, deciding on the timing and type of treatment intervention poses a significant challenge. The decision to treat should be based on symptom bother and the risk of complications whilst the therapeutic aims are to improve detrusor contractility, decrease Bladder outlet obstruction (BOO) or both. There is renewed interest in the development of pharmacotherapy to improve detrusor contractility, however there is a paucity of evidence in the published literature to support the widespread use of any agents. Therefore, the goal of managing the patient with DU is to optimise bladder emptying. This is most commonly achieved by conservative therapies, catheterisation, or surgery.

Clearly, the presence of a significantly raised post-voiding residual (PVR), which is associated with complications such as bladder stones, renal failure or recurrent urinary tract infections (UTI) would prompt consideration of treatment, although there is no evidence to suggest how many UTIs would prompt one to intervene. However, as the natural history of the disease is not completely understood; why some patients with DUA develop progression, while others do not, makes the decision of when and how to intervene in those without these 'absolute' indications more difficult. The limited available data suggests that the majority of men with DU show little evidence of progression as demonstrated in a study of 69 men with DU (as defined as Q_{max} <15 ml/s and P_{det} at Q_{max} of <40 cmH_2O), managed conservatively, where there was only minimal symptomatic progression or deterioration in urodynamic parameters over a 10 year period [1].

Symptom Scores and QoL

The use of patient reported outcome measures (PROM) and quality of life (QoL) scores are useful in the evaluation of lower urinary tract dysfunction and can demonstrate outcome following institution of treatments. However no validated PROM currently exists that is designed specifically for the diagnosis and follow-up of patients with DU. The IPSS and AUA-SI can be helpful, however there is a lack of emphasis on specific symptoms associated with DU and therefore novel PROMs are currently being developed [2]. In this study, the symptoms, which patients with DU predominantly complained of as compared to those with BOO included the sensation of incomplete emptying, urinary urgency and incontinence episodes. The development of PROMs, which are specific to DU will help to quantify the severity of symptoms and assess the response to treatment.

Conservative Treatment

In clinical practice, conservative measures have often already been instituted by the patient, with the aim of reducing the symptoms associated with incomplete emptying. For those with poor bladder sensation, scheduled voiding can reduce the number of urgency or incontinence episodes, while double voiding may act to ensure more complete bladder emptying thereby reducing the burden of urinary frequency. While specific expression techniques, such as the Crede's manoeuvre can be useful in some patients with neurogenic DU (and a weak outlet), it is not generally recommended due to the risk of producing high intra-vesical pressures, which can lead to vesico-ureteric reflux. Pelvic floor physiotherapy and biofeedback has been demonstrated to improve relaxation of the pelvic floor musculature, thereby reducing the outlet resistance and facilitating bladder emptying in patients with acontractile detrusors during conventional urodynamics [3] and women with dysfunctional voiding.

Catheterisation

It is generally accepted that patients with DU experience poorer outcomes after TURP [4] and many advocate the need for long term intermittent self catheterisation (ISC) or indwelling catheterisation. ISC is the preferred method for establishing bladder drainage in those with bothersome high PVRs, provided that manual dexterity, visual acuity and cognition are adequate. For those who are unwilling or incapable of performing ISC, long-term indwelling catheterisation is an option and a suprapubic catheter is clearly a better option than urethral catheterisation. Certainly, bladder drainage should be instituted in those who suffer with recurrent urinary tract infections associated with a significantly raised post-voiding residual, but it may also be appropriate for patients with DU who empty their bladder reasonably well but wish to speed up their voiding time by performing ISC, or those with bothersome urinary frequency or nocturia, where conservative management alone has failed.

Outlet Surgery

It has long been considered that DU occurs as a consequence of prolonged bladder outlet obstruction (BOO), an assumption that has largely been derived from *in vivo* studies using BOO models [5, 6]. Interestingly, in man there is little good evidence that this scenario is the case; in a cohort study by Thomas et al. [7], where 170 men with BOO were followed up over a 14 year period there was no significant deterioration in urodynamic parameters. Of men who decompensate acutely, i.e develop acute urinary retention, most would have preserved detrusor function, whilst many of those where the decompensation process is less acute (ie chronic retention) retain bladder contractility as seen in high-pressure chronic retention [8, 9]. This highlights the complex nature of pathophysiological mechanisms involved in the development of this condition. When considering outlet surgery in men with DU, categorisation into two clinical groups is relevant:

1. Those with DU, who empty their bladder relatively well and whose main complaint is symptoms.
2. Patients with DU who are catheter dependent (those referred to as having chronic urinary retention).

It is difficult to exclude the presence of a relative degree of BOO in the former group of patients on the basis of invasive urodynamics (due to the requirement of sufficient pressure to demonstrate BOO), however this is generally less likely to be of clinical significance, as these patients are able to empty their bladder with lower voiding pressures. Therefore, reducing outlet resistance (e.g. with a Transurethral resection of the prostate (TURP)) is unlikely to improve their symptoms; an assumption, which is supported by findings from Thomas et al. [10], where 22 men with DU underwent TURP, the majority of whom received surgery for symptoms only. There was no significant symptomatic benefit to these men, nor improvements in flow rate or voiding efficiency.

In the second clinical scenario, where the patient has DU and is catheter dependent, it is much more likely that the bladder has either undergone significant decompensation or there is a more significant BOO present. The goal of reducing outlet resistance in this context is to facilitate improved bladder emptying to get the patient catheter free. Although it is widely accepted that these patients do less well following TURP than those with confirmed BOO and preserved contractility [11], some do resume spontaneous voiding sufficient to empty their bladder to a significant degree [12]. Studies which have identified factors that are associated with a poorer outcome following TURP are summarised in Table 5.1. These predictors include low voiding detrusor pressures (<45 cmH_2O) [11], age >80 and a post voiding residual >1500 ml [9]. In the study by Ghalayini [11], recovery of voiding pressures were seen in patients (with a Pdetat Qmx >45 cmH_2O) following a period of ISC, suggesting that better outcomes could be expected following a TURP if ISC is performed pre-operatively. In the absence of other effective therapies, many surgeons will consider surgery younger men with DU, who are motivated to become catheter free. In such cases the importance of thorough pre-operative patient counselling cannot be over emphasized.

More recently, non-invasive markers of BOO, such as detrusor wall thickness (DWT) have come to the fore. Oelke et al. [13] demonstrated that the positive predictive value of a DWT of ≥2 mm for predicting BOO was 94 %. The clinical significance of this was demonstrated by Huang and co-authors, who suggested that a DWT <15 mm was associated with an unfavourable outcome after TURP [14] and that this could be a promising and helpful marker. It should be borne in mind however that these markers were primarily assessed for the diagnosis of BOO and their use for the diagnosis of DU has yet be established. Certainly the exclusion of a significant BOO by non invasive means could open the door for the instigation of DU pharmacotherapy or the basis of symptoms, uroflometry and PVR.

For women with DU, there is a paucity of evidence available in the literature to suggest a benefit for the routine use of urethral dilatation in such patients [15] and bladder neck incision in female patients should be avoided, as this can lead to incontinence or bladder neck contracture.

Conclusions

The available literature would suggest that for patients with DU, bladder emptying strategies should be implemented for those with recurrent urinary tract infec-

Table 5.1 Studies, which identify predictors of poorer outcome following TURP

Study	Population	Size	Mean age (range)	Diagnostic criteria	Outcomes	Predictor of poor outcome
Ghalayini et al. (2005) [11]	Men with chronic retention randomized to TURP or ISC	TURP 17 ISC 24	TURP 67 (52–84) ISC 69 (55–85)	IPSS >7 PVR >300	Improvement in IPSS, QoL, and PVR in both groups	Nine patients with Pdetat Qmax <45 had no significant improvement
Djavan et al. (1997) [9]	Men presenting with acute retention	81	72 (56–93)	Men with acute retention (without HPCR)	13 % failure after TURP, of whom: Mean age 84 versus 70 in success group Retention volume 1780 ml versus 1080 ml in success group Max Pdet (24 cmH_2O vs 74cmH_2O)	Age >80 PVR >1500 ml Absence of DOA

tions or bladder stones that are associated with a raised post voiding residual. This can be successfully achieved with ISC if it is a feasible option for patients. At present, pharmacotherapy directed at improving detrusor contractility is lacking an appropriate evidence base to suggest its widespread use in such patients. Outlet surgery is an option for men with DU who wish to be catheter-free; the outcomes following which are significantly poorer for men without significant BOO and several predictors of success have been proposed. These include a patient age <80, a Pdetat Qmax >45 cmH_2O and a PVR at presentation of <1500 ml. Given the difficulties associated with assessing for the presence of BOO in patients with DU, other methods for identifying the presence of BOO in this context have been proposed, such as the DWT. However this measurement has not yet been thoroughly assessed in the DU population.

References

1. Thomas AW, et al. The natural history of lower urinary tract dysfunction in men: minimum 10-year urodynamic follow-up of untreated detrusor underactivity. BJU Int. 2005;96(9): 1295–300.
2. Uren A, et al. The patient experience of underactive bladder. Eur Urol Suppl. 2016; 15(3):e995.
3. van Koeveringe GA, Rahnama'i MS, Berghmans BC. The additional value of ambulatory urodynamic measurements compared with conventional urodynamic measurements. BJU Int. 2010;105(4):508–13.
4. Dubey D, et al. Acute urinary retention: defining the need and timing for pressure-flow studies. BJU Int. 2001;88(3):178–82.
5. Levin RM, et al. Studies on experimental bladder outlet obstruction in the cat: long-term functional effects. J Urol. 1992;148(3):939–43.
6. Saito M, et al. Effects of partial outflow obstruction on bladder contractility and blood flow to the detrusor: comparison between mild and severe obstruction. Urol Int. 1997;59(4): 226–30.
7. Thomas AW, et al. The natural history of lower urinary tract dysfunction in men: minimum 10-year urodynamic follow-up of untreated bladder outlet obstruction. BJU Int. 2005;96(9):1301–6.
8. George NJ, et al. High pressure chronic retention. Br Med J (Clin Res Ed). 1983;286(6380): 1780–3.
9. Djavan B, et al. Urodynamic assessment of patients with acute urinary retention: is treatment failure after prostatectomy predictable? J Urol. 1997;158(5):1829–33.
10. Thomas AW, et al. The natural history of lower urinary tract dysfunction in men: the influence of detrusor underactivity on the outcome after transurethral resection of the prostate with a minimum 10-year urodynamic follow-up. BJU Int. 2004;93(6):745–50.
11. Ghalayini IF, Al-Ghazo MA, Pickard RS. A prospective randomized trial comparing transurethral prostatic resection and clean intermittent self-catheterization in men with chronic urinary retention. BJU Int. 2005;96(1):93–7.
12. Monoski MA, et al. Urodynamic predictors of outcomes with photoselective laser vaporization prostatectomy in patients with benign prostatic hyperplasia and preoperative retention. Urology. 2006;68(2):312–7.

13. Oelke M, et al. Diagnostic accuracy of noninvasive tests to evaluate bladder outlet obstruction in men: detrusor wall thickness, uroflowmetry, postvoid residual urine, and prostate volume. Eur Urol. 2007;52(3):827–34.
14. Huang T, et al. Predictive value of resistive index, detrusor wall thickness and ultrasound estimated bladder weight regarding the outcome after transurethral prostatectomy for patients with lower urinary tract symptoms suggestive of benign prostatic obstruction. Int J Urol. 2012;19(4):343–50.
15. Basu M, Duckett J. The effect of urethral dilatation on pressure flow studies in women with voiding dysfunction and overactive bladder. Int Urogynecol J Pelvic Floor Dysfunct. 2009;20(9):1073–7.

Pharmacological Treatment of Underactive Bladder

6

K.E. Andersson

Key Points

- Underactive bladder (UAB) and detrusor underactivity (DUA) are difficult to treat pharmacologically due to their multifactorial pathophysiology
- Theoretically, these conditions can be improved by agents that increase detrusor contractile activity and decrease bladder capacity, and/or decrease outlet resistance
- However, current treatments, including muscarinic receptor agonists, such as bethanechol and carbachol, choline esterase inhibitors, like distigmine, and α1-adrenoceptor antagonists, have limited efficacy
- Since the pathophysiology of UAB/DUA, involving both central and peripheral factors, may be complicated, successful therapy has to be directed to both the major mechanism involved and to the associated morbidities.

Introduction

As discussed elsewhere [1–4] the Underactive Bladder (UAB: symptom diagnosis) and Detrusor Underactivity (DUA: urodynamic diagnosis) have multifactorial pathophysiologies, which introduce obvious therapeutic problems. Not only can the pathophysiologies vary between patients, but also in an individual patient several factors may contribute, and it is not always possible to identify "major" and "minor"

K.E. Andersson, MD, PhD
Institute for Regenerative Medicine, Wake Forest University School of Medicine, Winston Salem, NC, USA

Institute of Clinical Medicine, Department of Obstetrics and Gynecology, Aarhus University Hospital, Palle Juul-Jensens Boulevard 99, DK 8200 Aarhus N, Denmark
e-mail: Keanders@wakehealth.edu

C.R. Chapple et al. (eds.), *Underactive Bladder*,
DOI 10.1007/978-3-319-43087-4_6

players that can be targets for treatment. Since complete bladder emptying is dependent on an intact central nervous system (CNS) control, normal sensation and detrusor smooth muscle activity, coordinated bladder and urethral sphincter function, and voluntary initiation of voiding, incomplete bladder emptying and urinary retention can result from disturbances of any of these components. If there are irreversible changes at any level, e.g., in the bladder wall (loss of nerves, loss of muscle tissue, increased collagen deposition), the possibilities of successful pharmacological treatment are reduced.

"Detrusor Hyperactivity with Impaired Contractility" (DHIC: [5]) is a diagnosis related to both overactive bladder (OAB)/detrusor overactivity (DO) and UAB/DUA, and the condition creates therapeutic challenges. However, as pointed out by several investigators, UAB/DUA and OAB/DO may not be separate disease entities [6–9]. Instead, chronic untreated or treatment-refractory OAB/DO, caused by neurologic diseases, diabetes, BOO, ischemic bladder dysfunction, or aging, may progress to DO with impaired contractility and eventually to UAB/DU. Progression of OAB/DO to UAB/DUA has been demonstrated in animal models [9, 10] and, if proven also in humans, suggests that early education, behavioral modification, and medical treatment may alter and/or prevent progression to UAB/DUA [7].

To what extent drug treatment of associated morbidities (e.g., diabetes, Parkinson's disease, multiple sclerosis) also can improve impaired bladder emptying has only been investigated to a limited extent.

Pharmacological Principles Used for Treatment

To improve bladder emptying, agents that increase the contractile force of the detrusor, decrease outflow resistance, or improve detrusor contractility and decrease outflow resistance at the same time, would theoretically be useful [11]. In addition, agents that improve decreased sensation (increase afferent activity and/or the perception of bladder filling) seem attractive [12]. However, in many cases the pathophysiology of UAB/DUA is complex, simultaneously involving several mechanisms [1–4]. This implies that targeting only one potentially important mechanism will not always have the desired effect.

Muscarinic Receptor Agonists and Cholinesterase Inhibitors

It is well established the acetylcholine is the main contractile transmitter in the detrusor muscle, and that release of this agent induced by activation of the parasympathetic outflow from the spinal cord leads to a co-ordinated bladder contraction and bladder emptying with simultaneous relaxation of the outflow region [13]. Standard pharmacotherapy of impaired bladder emptying has for a long time included muscarinic receptor agonists, such as bethanechol and carbachol to directly stimulate muscarinic receptors on the detrusor muscle, or choline esterase inhibitors, like distigmine to reduce the degradation of acetylcholine. However, based on available information it has been considered that little, if any, beneficial effects can be obtained in preventing or treating UAB/DUA [14, 15]. Why do these drugs not work? One of the reasons is that direct stimulation of detrusor muscarinic receptors will cause contraction of the bladder without simultaneous relaxation of the outflow region. Activation of the cholinergic nerves of the outflow region by spinal parasympathetic outflow will not only release acetylcholine for bladder contraction, but also nitric oxide, relaxing the urethra. Injection of non-subtype muscarinic receptor agonists such as bethanechol and carbachol will cause a "contracture" of both bladder and urethra, and cause a transient increase in intravesical pressure. This may possibly trigger a micturition reflex and emptying of the bladder, but this effect seems unreliable. In addition, systemic administration of muscarinic receptor agonists has no selectivity for the bladder which means that action on non-target sites will cause adverse effects. Another factor is that both bethanechol and carbachol have low oral bioavailability which makes it difficult to attain "active" blood concentrations.

Bethanechol seems to be the best investigated of the parasympathomimetic drugs. Even if beneficial effects have been reported, most studies have shown no significant effect vs placebo in the treatment of UAB/DUA Barendrecht et al. [14]. Attempts have been made to increase the usefulness of muscarinic agonist stimulation. Riedl et al. [16] used electromotive administration of intravesical bethanechol and could identify patients with an atonic bladder and adequate residual detrusor muscle function. They concluded that patients who do not respond to the electromotive administration of bethanechol do not benefit from oral bethanechol and are candidates for catheterization. To combine bladder contraction and outflow relaxation,

Hindley et al. [17], in a placebo-controlled study, treated 19 patients with DUA with a combination of intravesical PGE_2 and oral bethanechol. They concluded that there was evidence of a pharmacological effect with a limited therapeutic efficacy compared with placebo. However, this treatment was not recommended as routine, but only for the occasional treatment of a patient with DUA. In summary, available information shows that the beneficial effects that can be obtained with carbachol and bethanechol in preventing or treating UAB/DUA are small or negligible [14, 15].

A number of studies have tested the effect of distigmine bromide on voiding efficiency, but the results have been conflicting. In a double-blind study, Shah et al. [18] investigated the effect of distigmine bromide versus placebo on voiding after prostatectomy 93 patients. The results showed a trend towards improvement, but no statistically significant increase in post-operative flow rates, in reduction in bladder volume, and in the incidence of re-catheterisation in the patients treated with the drug. In a prospective randomized study on 100 patients undergoing vaginal surgery for genital prolapse, Savona Ventura et al. [19] compared distigmine bromide, phenoxybenzamine hydrochloride, and prostaglandin $F_{2\alpha}$, to prevent urinary retention. They found that all agents appeared to increase the incidence of an elevated residual urinary volume by about three times. Even if the mechanisms behind these findings are difficult to explain, they clearly do not encourage the use of these agents on the indication.

Philp and Thomas [20] gave distigmine bromide to 23 patients with paraplegia due to suprasacral spinal cord injury who retained a reflex micturition. There was a marked reduction of the residual urine volume in all patients whilst being on parenteral distigmine. The oral preparation of the drug proved less effective and this was attributed to poor absorption from the gut. Tanaka et al. [21] found in 14 patients with poor detrusor contractility after transurethral prostatectomy (TURP) that oral administration of distigmine bromide (5 mg three times daily for 4 weeks) resulted in subjective as well as objective improvement; the International Prostate Symptom Score (IPSS) was reduced from a mean of 18.9 to a mean of <10 and the maximum flow increased from a mean of 8.9 ml/s to a mean of >12 ml/s. In addition, detrusor contractility tended to improve. Bougas et al. [22] investigated 27 patients (11 men and 16 women) with poor detrusor function established using pressure-flow studies. They were treated with distigmine bromide for 4 weeks which resulted in a statistically significant reduction of residual volume (from a mean of 329.1 to a mean of 156.8 ml), obviating the need for intermittent self-catheterisation in 11 patients. In addition, maximum flow rate and detrusor pressure at maximum flow increased, although not significantly. The drug was generally well tolerated by the majority of patients.

It is obvious that the most positive effects of distigmine have been obtained in non-placebo controlled studies with small patient materials with various diagnoses. It cannot be excluded that in some selected patient categories distigmine may have a positive effect, but the lack of adequately designed studies implies that a fair assessment of the drug as a general treatment of UAB/DUA is not possible.

In a recent, open, non-randomized pilot study on 19 patients with DUA, Sugimoto et al. [23] studied the effects of acotiamide, a drug approved in Japan for treatment various gastrointestinal disorders [24]. Acotiamide "appears to exert an antagonistic effect on muscarinic M1, M2, and M3 receptors and thereby inhibit the negative feedback system by blocking muscarinic auto receptors that regulate acetylcholine release." The main outcome parameter of the study was post-void residual (PVR) which after acotiamide changed from 161.4 ± 90.0 mL at baseline to 116.3 ± 63.1 mL at 2- weeks post-treatment. This may be statistically significant but is not very impressive. If the mechanism of action of the drug is increased acetylcholine release, it may not differ from other parasympathomimetic drugs.

Currently used parasympathomimetic agents are often administered in doses too low to be effective on the detrusor. A reason for underdosing could be a fear of side-effects, e.g., flushing, nausea, vomiting, diarrhoea, gastrointestinal cramps, bronchospasms, headache, salivation, sweating, and difficulty with visual accommodation. Rare but important side-effects include acute and severe cardiovascular depression, which can result in an acute circulatory failure and cardiac arrest and hence be potentially lethal [14].

For all parasympathomimetic drugs, well-designed, randomized controlled trials on well-defined patient materials are lacking, implying that these drugs cannot be recommended for general use, but may potentially be utilized for personalized treatment of UAB/DUA.

α-Adrenoceptor Antagonists

The role of α-adrenoceptor (AR) antagonists in the treatment of voiding symptoms in men with bladder outflow obstruction (BOO) is well documented [25, 26] Although most men with voiding symptoms do not necessarily have UAB/DUA, the drugs may improve bladder emptying in these patients. Supporting this, α_1- AR antagonists have been widely used in the conservative management of acute urinary retention caused by BOO as shown in a recent systematic review and meta-analysis of available data [27].

In patients with neurogenic bladder, reduction of urethral resistance during voiding by α-AR antagonists have been reported to be useful [28–33]. However, most of the studies have been performed on small patient materials with varying diagnoses and all studies have not been positive. In a study of 14 children from age 6 to 16 years with neurogenic bladder and LPP > 40 cm H_2O, Kroll et al. [34] found no evident efficacy of doxazosin after 6–8 weeks of treatment. Yamanishi et al. [35] reported in a prospective single-blind randomized study that the combination of a cholinergic drug (bethanechol) and a α_1- AR antagonist (urapidil) was more effective than monotherapy in improving urination in patients with UAB/DUA. Theoretically, the approach of enhancing detrusor contractility and lowering urethral resistance simultaneously seems attractive. However, in the study by Yamanishi et al. (2004), monotherapy with bethanechol seemed to be marginal, and whether the combination therapy really is better than monotherapy with α-AR antagonist has to be confirmed in appropriately designed studies.

Prostanoids

Previous experimental studies have shown that e.g., prostaglandin (PG) E_2 can both increase detrusor contraction and relax the urethra in humans [36]. PGE_2 does not only stimulate detrusor contraction directly, but may also enhance the efficacy of other contraction-mediating transmitters. In addition, PGE_2 can increase afferent activity both by stimulating the urothelial and myogenic pathways [37, 38].

Intravesical instillation of PGE2 and other prostanoids has been reported (no controlled randomized trials) to stimulate bladder contractile activity acutely [39–42], but not without side effects (e.g., uterine contraction). Experiences from patients with chronic bladder emptying difficulties [43] or neurogenic bladder dysfunction [44] have not been encouraging. The question is whether useful actions can be sorted out from the mixture of effects exerted by PGE_2. The effects of this prostanoid are produced through four types of EP-receptors (EP1-EP4), each mediating separate actions [45]. EP1 and EP3 receptors seem to mediate the excitatory bladder effects of PGE_2 both on afferent activity and on smooth muscle, and EP2 receptors are known to mediate bladder and urethral relaxation. Drugs stimulating both EP3 and EP2 receptors simultaneously would have an interesting profile, and provided that they show selectivity for the bladder over e.g., the uterus and the gastrointestinal tract, they should be interesting to test in patients with UAB. ONO-8055 is a highly potent and selective agonist for both EP2 and EP3 receptors on Chines Hamster Ovary (CHO) cells) [46]. The compound contracted bladder strips and relaxed urethral strips. Awake cystometry in a model of neurogenic bladder (lumbar spinal stenosis) showed that ONO-8055 significantly decreased bladder capacity, residual urine, and voiding pressure. Compared with the vehicle, tamsulosin and ONO-8055 significantly decreased urethral pressure. The authors concluded that ONO-8055 had potential to ameliorate neurogenic UAB/DUA. However, to prove this controlled clinical trials are required.

Transient Receptor Potential (TRP) Channel Agonists

TRP channels are widely distributed in the LUT and stimulation and blockade of these channels may have a potential application for treatment of various voiding disturbances, including UAB/DUA [47–52]. Agents such as capsaicin and resiniferatoxin stimulate bladder activity via activation of Transient Receptor Potential (TRP) channel V1 [53]. This should make small molecule TRPV1 agonists an interesting future option for treatment of UAB/DUA, provided that they do not desensitize the afferent nerves.

TRPM4 channels seem to regulate human detrusor smooth muscle excitability and contractility and are critical determinants of human urinary bladder function, actions that may be worthwhile exploring [54].

Even if the pharmacological profile of some of the TRP channel active drugs (based on preclinical studies) seem promising for treatment of UAB/DUA, which agent (s) to choose for further development remains speculative since there are no published clinical experiences.

5-Hydroxytryptamine (Serotonin)

Many preclinical studies have shown serotonin, acting on a variety of receptor subtypes both peripherally and on the central nervous system, to have diverse effects on micturition [55]. If some of these effects were valid also for humans, they would have potential interest for the treatment of UAB/DUA [55]. Serotonin has a well-established contractile effect on human bladder strips mediated by 5-HT4 receptors via facilitation of cholinergic neuromuscular transmission [56, 57], and an occasional case report suggests efficacy in some cases of UAB/DUA with cisapride [58], a 5-HT4 agonist with 5-HT3 antagonist activity,widely used to promote gastrointestinal motility, but withdrawn because of cardiac (long QT) side effects [59]. Whether or not analogues without this side effect would be useful can only be speculated on.

Botulinum Toxin

Kuo [60] treated 27 patients with idiopathic low detrusor contractility with urethral injection of onabotulinum A toxin (BoNT-A). It was found that patients with normal bladder sensation combined with a poor relaxation or hyperactive urethral sphincter were significantly more likely to recover normal detrusor function. Further studies on such patients would be desirable.

Conclusions

The current pharmacological possibilities to effectively treat UAB/DUA are limited. Dependent on the multifactorial pathophysiology of the condition, treatment with approved agents has to be personalized and to be successful therapy has to be directed to both the major mechanism involved and the associated morbidities.

References

1. Andersson KE. The many faces of impaired bladder emptying. Curr Opin Urol. 2014;24(4):363–9.
2. Miyazato M, Yoshimura N, Chancellor MB. The other bladder syndrome: underactive bladder. Rev Urol. 2013;15(1):11–22.
3. Osman NI, Chapple CR, Abrams P, Dmochowski R, Haab F, Nitti V, Koelbl H, van Kerrebroeck P, Wein AJ. Detrusor underactivity and the underactive bladder: a new clinical entity? A review of current terminology, definitions, epidemiology, aetiology, and diagnosis. Eur Urol. 2014;65(2):389–98.
4. Osman NI, Chapple CR. Contemporary concepts in the aetiopathogenesis of detrusor underactivity. Nat Rev Urol. 2014;11(11):639–48.
5. Resnick NM, Yalla SV. Detrusor hyperactivity with impaired contractile function. An unrecognized but common cause of incontinence in elderly patients. JAMA. 1987;257(22): 3076–81.
6. Semins MJ, Chancellor MB. Diagnosis and management of patients with overactive bladder syndrome and abnormal detrusor activity. Nat Clin Pract Urol. 2004;1(2):78–84.
7. Chancellor MB. The overactive bladder progression to underactive bladder hypothesis. Int Urol Nephrol. 2014;46 Suppl 1:S23–7.
8. Liu Z, Uchiyama T, Sakakibara R, Yamamoto T. Underactive and overactive bladders are related to motor function and quality of life in Parkinson's disease. Int Urol Nephrol. 2015;47(5):751–7.
9. Nomiya M, Yamaguchi O, Akaihata H, Hata J, Sawada N, Kojima Y, Andersson KE. Progressive vascular damage may lead to bladder underactivity in rats. J Urol. 2014;191(5):1462–9.
10. Nomiya M, Miyazaki N, Ikegami K, Yamaguchi O. Bladder overactivity may progress to bladder underactivity in a rat model of chronic bladder ischemia. Montreal: ICS; 2015.
11. Wein AJ. Pathophysiology and categorization of voiding dysfunction. In: Walsh PC, Retik AB, Vaughan ED, Wein AJ, editors. Campbell's urology, vol. 2. 8th ed. Philadelphia: W.B. Saunders; 2002. p. 887–99.
12. Smith PP, Chalmers DJ, Feinn RS. Does defective volume sensation contribute to detrusor underactivity? Neurourol Urodyn. 2015;34(8):752–6.
13. Andersson KE, Arner A. Urinary bladder contraction and relaxation: physiology and pathophysiology. Physiol Rev. 2004;84(3):935–86.

14. Barendrecht MM, Oelke M, Laguna MP, Michel MC. Is the use of parasympathomimetics for treating an underactive urinary bladder evidence-based? BJU Int. 2007;99(4):749.
15. Andersson KE, Chapple CR, Cardozo L, Cruz F, Gratzke C, Lee KS, Tannenbaum C, Wein AJ. Chapter 8: Pharmacological treatment of urinary incontinence. In: Abrams P, Cardozo L, Khoury S, Wein AJ, editors. Incontinence. 5th ed. 5th international consultation on incontinence, Paris, February, 2012, ICUD-EAU 2013. p. 623–728
16. Riedl CR, Stephen RL, Daha LK, Knoll M, Plas E, Pflüger H. Electromotive administration of intravesical bethanechol and the clinical impact on acontractile detrusor management: introduction of a new test. J Urol. 2000;164(6):2108–11.
17. Hindley RG, Brierly RD, Thomas PJ. Prostaglandin E2 and bethanechol in combination for treating detrusorunderactivity. BJU Int. 2004;93(1):89–92.
18. Shah PJ, Abrams PH, Choa RG, Ashken MH, Gaches CG, Green NA, Wiles A. Distigmine bromide and post prostatectomy voiding. Br J Urol. 1983;55:229–32.
19. Savona-Ventura C, Grech ES, Saliba I. Pharmacological measures to prevent post-operative urinary retention; a prospective randomized study. Eur J Obstet Gynecol Reprod Biol. 1991;41:225–9.
20. Philp NH, Thomas DG. The effect of distigmine bromide on voiding in male paraplegic patients with reflex micturition. Br J Urol. 1980;52(6):492–6.
21. Tanaka Y, Masumori N, Itoh N, Furuya S, Nishizawa O, Tsukamoto T. Symptomatic and urodynamic improvement by oral distigmine bromide in poor voiders after transurethral resection of the prostate. Urology. 2001;57(2):270–4.
22. Bougas DA, Mitsogiannis IC, Mitropoulos DN, Kollaitis GC, Serafetinides EN, Giannopoulos AM. Clinical efficacy of distigmine bromide in the treatment of patients with underactive detrusor. Int Urol Nephrol. 2004;36(4):507–12.
23. Sugimoto K, Akiyama T, Shimizu N, Matsumura N, Hayashi T, Nishioka T, Uemura H. A pilot study of acotiamide hydrochloride hydrate in patients with detrusor underactivity. Res Rep Urol. 2015;7:81–3.
24. Doi Y, Murasaki O, Kaibara M, Uezono Y, Hayashi H, Yano K, Taniyama K. Characterization of functional effects of Z-338, a novel gastroprokinetic agent, on the muscarinic M1, M2, and M3 receptors expressed in Xenopus oocytes. Eur J Pharmacol. 2004;505(1–3):31–5.
25. Michel MC. The forefront for novel therapeutic agents based on the pathophysiology of lower urinary tract dysfunction: alpha-blockers in the treatment of male voiding dysfunction - how do they work and why do they differ in tolerability? J Pharmacol Sci. 2010;112(2):151–7.
26. Lepor H, Kazzazi A, Djavan B. α-Blockers for benign prostatic hyperplasia: the new era. Curr Opin Urol. 2012;22(1):7–15.
27. Guang-Jun D, Feng-Bin G, Xun-Bo J. A_1-blockers in the management of acute urinary retention secondary to benign prostatic hyperplasia: a systematic review and meta-analysis. Ir J Med Sci. 2015;184(1):23–30.
28. Mobley DF. Phenoxybenzamine in the management of neurogenic vesical dysfunction. J Urol. 1976;116:737–8.
29. O'Riordan JI, Doherty C, Javed M, Brophy D, Hutchinson M, Quinlan D. Do a-blockers have a role in lower urinary tract dysfunction in multiple sclerosis? J Urol. 1995;153:1114–6.
30. Sakakibara R, Hattori T, Uchiyama T, Suenaga T, Takahashi H, Yamanishi T, Egoshi K, Sekita N. Are alphablockers involved in lower urinary tract dysfunction in multiple system atrophy? A comparison of prazosin and moxisylyte. J Auton Nerv Syst. 2000;79:191–5.
31. Schulte-Baukloh H, Michael T, Miller K, Knispel HH. Alfuzosin in the treatment of high leak-point pressure in children with neurogenic bladder. BJU Int. 2002;90:716–20.
32. Yamanishi T, Yasuda K, Homma Y, Kawabe K, Morita T. A multicenter placebo-controlled, double-blind trial of urapidil, an α-blocker, on neurogenic bladder dysfunction. Eur Urol. 1999;35:45–51.
33. Moon KH, Park CH, Jung HC, Oh TH, Kim JS, Kim DY. A 12-week, open label, multi-center study to evaluate the clinical efficacy and safety of silodosin on voiding dysfunction in patients with neurogenic bladder. Low Urin Tract Symptoms. 2015;7(1):27–31.

34. Kroll P, Gajewska E, Zachwieja J, Sobieska M, Mańkowski P. An evaluation of the efficacy of selective alpha-blockers in the treatment of children with neurogenic bladder dysfunction-preliminary findings. Int J Environ Res Public Health. 2016;15:13(3).
35. Yamanishi T, Yasuda K, Kamai T, Tsujii T, Sakakibara R, Uchiyama T, Yoshida K. Combination of a cholinergic drug and an alpha-blocker is more effective than monotherapy for the treatment of voiding difficulty in patients with underactive detrusor. Int J Urol. 2004;11(2):88–96.
36. Andersson KE, Wein AJ. Pharmacology of the lower urinary tract: basis for current and future treatments of urinary incontinence. Pharmacol Rev. 2004;56(4):581–631.
37. Maggi CA, Giuliani S, Conte B, Furio M, Santicioli P, Meli P, Gragnani L, Meli A. Prostanoids modulate reflex micturition by acting through capsaicin-sensitive afferents. Eur J Pharmacol. 1988;145(2):105–12.
38. Maggi CA, Evangelista S, Grimaldi G, Santicioli P, Giolitti A, Meli A. Evidence for the involvement of arachidonic acid metabolites in spontaneous and drug-induced contractions of rat urinary bladder. J Pharmacol Exp Ther. 1984;230(2):500–13.
39. Andersson KE, Henriksson L, Ulmsten U. Effects of prostaglandin E2 applied locally on intravesical and intraurethral pressures in women. Eur Urol. 1978;4(5):366–9.
40. Wagner G, Husslein P, Enzelsberger H. Is prostaglandin E2 really of therapeutic value for postoperative urinary retention? Results of a prospectively randomized double-blind study. Am J Obstet Gynecol. 1985;151(3):375–9.
41. Tammela T, Kontturi M, Käär K, Lukkarinen O. Intravesical prostaglandin F2 for promoting bladder emptying after surgery for female stress incontinence. Br J Urol. 1987;60(1): 43–6.
42. Schüssler B. Comparison of the mode of action of prostaglandin E2 (PGE2) and sulprostone, a PGE2-derivative, on the lower urinary tract in healthy women. A urodynamic study. Urol Res. 1990;18(5):349–52.
43. Delaere KP, Thomas CM, Moonen WA, Debruyne FM. The value of intravesical instillation of 15(S)-15 methyl prostaglandin F2-alpha in patients with neurogenic bladder dysfunction. Br J Urol. 1981;53(4):306–9.
44. Vaidyanathan S, Rao MS, Mapa MK, Bapna BC, Chary KS, Swamy RP. Study of intravesical instillation of 15(S)-15 methyl prostaglandin F2-alpha in patients with neurogenic bladder dysfunction. J Urol. 1981;126(1):81–5.
45. Sugimoto Y, Narumiya S. Prostaglandin E receptors. Biol Chem. 2007;282(16):11613–7.
46. Sekido N, Kida J, Mashimo H, Wakamatsu D, Okada H, Matsuya H. Promising Effects of a Novel EP2 and EP3 Receptor Dual Agonist, ONO-8055, on Neurogenic Underactive Bladder in a Rat Lumbar Canal Stenosis Model. J Urol. 2016;196(2):609–16.
47. Everaerts W, Gevaert T, Nilius B, De Ridder D. On the origin of bladder sensing: tr(i)ps in urology. Neurourol Urodyn. 2008;27:264–73.
48. Andersson KE, Gratzke C, Hedlund P. The role of the transient receptor potential (TRP) superfamily of cation-selective channels in the management of the overactive bladder. BJU Int. 2010;106(8):1114–27.
49. Skryma R, Prevarskaya N, Gkika D, Shuba Y. From urgency to frequency: facts and controversies of TRPs in the lower urinary tract. Nat Rev Urol. 2011;8:617–30.
50. Avelino A, Charrua A, Frias B, Cruz C, Boudes M, de Ridder D, et al. Transient receptor potential channels in bladder function. Acta Physiol. 2013;207:110–22.
51. Franken J, Uvin P, De Ridder D, Voets T. TRP channels in lower urinary tract dysfunction. Br J Pharmacol. 2014;171:2537–51.
52. Deruyver Y, Voets T, De Ridder D, Everaerts W. Transient receptor potential channel modulators as pharmacological treatments for lower urinary tract symptoms: myth or reality? BJU Int. 2015;115:686–97.
53. Maggi CA, Barbanti G, Santicioli P, Beneforti P, Misuri D, Meli A, Turini D. Cystometric evidence that capsaicin-sensitive nerves modulate the afferent branch of micturition reflex in humans. J Urol. 1989;142(1):150–4.

54. Hristov KL, Smith AC, Parajuli SP, Malysz J, Rovner ES, Petkov GV. Novel regulatory mechanism in human urinary bladder: central role of transient receptor potential melastatin 4 channels in detrusor smooth muscle function. Am J Physiol Cell Physiol. 2016;310(7):C600–11.
55. Ramage AG. The role of central 5-hydroxytryptamine (5-HT, serotonin) receptors in the control of micturition. Br J Pharmacol. 2006;147 Suppl 2:S120–31.
56. Tonini M, Messori E, Franceschetti GP, Rizzi CA, Castoldi AF, Coccini T, Candura SM. Characterization of the 5-HT receptor potentiating neuromuscular cholinergic transmission in strips of human isolated detrusor muscle. Br J Pharmacol. 1994;113(1):1–2.
57. Candura SM, Messori E, Franceschetti GP, D'Agostino G, Vicini D, Tagliani M, Tonini M. Neural 5-HT4 receptors in the human isolated detrusor muscle: effects of indole, benzimidazolone and substituted benzamide agonists and antagonists. Br J Pharmacol. 1996; 118(8):1965–70.
58. Franceschetti GP, Candura SM, Vicini D, Tonini M. Cisapride enhances detrusor contractility and improves micturition in a woman with lazy bladder. Scand J Urol Nephrol. 1997; 31(2):209–10.
59. Quigley EM. Cisapride: what can we learn from the rise and fall of a prokinetic? J Dig Dis. 2011;12(3):147–56.
60. Kuo HC. Recovery of detrusor function after urethral botulinum a toxin injection in patients with idiopathic low detrusor contractility and voiding dysfunction. Urology. 2007;69(1): 57–61.

Surgical Treatment: Outlet Reduction, Men and Women

7

Bilal Chughtai, Dominique Thomas, Austin Te, and Steven A. Kaplan

Key Points

1. The most relevant preoperative test to determine the relative degree of DU and bladder outlet obstruction is a pressure flow urodynamic study, however the factors that predict outcome are not well characterized
2. For men outlet reduction, including TURP, HoLEP and PVP, has resulted in variable success in patients with DU.
3. The decision as to whether to perform surgical therapy in patients with DU should be highly individualized and include appropriate counseling as to the unpredictability of the outcome.
4. In absence of any demonstrable anatomical obstruction, there is currently no clear role for outlet reduction surgery in women with DU.

Introduction

The International Continence Society (ICS) defines detrusor underactivity (DU) as "a contraction of reduced strength and/or duration, resulting in prolonged bladder emptying and/or failure to achieve complete bladder emptying within normal time span" [1]. DU is thus a urodynamic diagnosis [2] which occurs in almost 48 % of older men (>65) and 13 % of older women (>65) evaluated for lower urinary tract symptoms (LUTS) [4]. DU can occur in association with chronic bladder outlet

B. Chughtai • D. Thomas • A. Te
Department of Urology, Weill Cornell Medicine,
425 East 61st Street, New York, NY 10065, USA
e-mail: bic9008@med.cornell.edu; dot2007@med.cornell.edu; agt29@cornell.edu

S.A. Kaplan, M.D (✉)
Professor of Urology, Icahn School of Medicine at Mount Sinai, New York, NY, USA
e-mail: steven.kaplan@mountsinai.org

C.R. Chapple et al. (eds.), *Underactive Bladder*,
DOI 10.1007/978-3-319-43087-4_7

obstruction, aging, myogenic or various neurogenic defects or idiopathic causes [2]. Clinically DU is characterized by voiding LUTS and reduced voiding efficiency [3]. DU is also associated with complications such as recurrent urinary tract infections and bladder stones.

Urodynamics are essential in the determination of the relative contribution of bladder outlet resistance and DU to patients' symptoms. This is particularly important when considering surgery to the bladder outlet. There has however been a lack of literature regarding the urodynamic evaluation of DU [5]. Clearly preoperative planning, extensive patient counselling are necessary before any surgical procedure in this cohort. The aim of this chapter is to provide an analysis of the role of outlet reduction surgery in both men and women with underlying DU.

Pre-operative Studies

The most useful test to determine the degree of BOO and detrusor contractility is a pressure flow urodynamic study [6]. In addition important information such as bladder sensation, compliance and capacity that is relevant to preoperative planning can also be gleaned [6]. Several urodynamic measures of bladder contractility are described and are described in detail in Chap. 3 . Estimation of post-void residual (PVR) with the use of ultrasound or catheterization is essential to determine to voiding efficiency. A synchronous videourodynamic study (VUDS) may provide valuable insight on the degree and nature of bladder outlet obstruction [7]. It is important to keep in mind that a major limitation in the use of more traditional methods for urodynamics when diagnosing DU compared to BOO is that when diagnosing BOO it is highly dependent on the degree of bladder contractility ref.

Outlet Reduction Surgery for Men

Transurethral Resection of the Prostate (TURP)

TURP is the gold standard when treating LUTS secondary to benign prostatic hyperplasia (BPH). There is limited data on patients with DU undergoing TURP. Tanaka et al. conducted a clinical study to evaluate the short-term efficacy of TURP on BOO, DO and DU. They recruited 92 males over the age of 50 who were considered suitable candidates for the procedure [10]. Patients underwent preoperative pressure flow study analyses before undergoing TURP. Overall, TURP demonstrated a 76 % overall efficacy rate amongst patients [10]. From baseline to 3-months follow-up patients showed improvements in all parameters across all degrees of bladder outlet obstruction based on linPURR scores. Furthermore, it was markedly higher amongst patients with BOO as these levels worsened, while TURP had no significant benefit on those with DU or DO [10]. In conclusion, 20 % of those with DU achieved good efficacy after undergoing TURP. IPSS scores for those with weak/very weak detrusor contractility at 3-months after TURP improved from 14.8 to 4.7, $p<0.001$. Qmax improved from 10.8 to 18.9 mL/s, $p<0.001$ and PVR decreased from 47.1 to 24.3, $p<0.001$ 3-month after TURP.

Masumori et al. evaluated whether DU could potentially affect the long-term outcomes of TURP. Of the original 92 patients in the study by Tanaka et al., 34 were eligible to continue in the study. Those with DU that IPSS scores improved by 3-months post procedure, but degraded over time (3-months 5.2 vs. 12 years 10.1) [9]. This was similarly seen for QoL (3-months 1.8 vs. 12 years 2.2). Interestingly, despite poor objective results, 2/3 of patients diagnosed with DU reported being content with their current urinary symptoms [9].

Thomas et al. evaluated the outcome of TURP in men with DU [11]. In a cohort of 224 men who had been diagnosed with DU, 22 patients had undergone TURP. The rest of the cohort was treated with clean intermittent catheterization (CIC) or watchful waiting [11]. The authors showed a long-term reduction in obstruction as evaluated through detrusor pressure at Qmax (pdetQmax = baseline 31 vs. follow-up 25, $p=0.027$) and BOO index (BOOI = baseline 15 vs. follow-up 9, $p=0.029$) [11]. When compared to those who did not undergo any formal treatment, patients who underwent TURP did not show any significant urodynamic differences. Interestingly those who underwent TURP showed a statistically significant decrease in bladder voiding efficiency (BVE) for which there is no apparent explanation [11]. Those not undergoing any treatment who were followed up had a BVE = 82 compared to a BVE = 58 ($p=0.044$) in those who underwent TURP [11]. The authors concluded DU is a contraindication for TURP.

Although, patients with DU undergoing TURP do not seem to derive much benefit based on objective urodynamic parameters, there is some evidence of patient satisfaction following the procedure. Overall there is a paucity of information available to make any firm recommendation as to which patients with DU should undergo TURP and case by case approach is advocated.

Laser Prostatectomy

An alternative method of reducing outlet resistance is the transurethral laser prostatectomy. Laser prostatectomy differs from TURP by "delivering heat to the prostatic tissue through a laser fiber under cystoscopic vision" [12]. As with TURP, there is a limited number of published studies examining its effect on patients with DU. Currently, laser prostatectomy is performed with several different lasers such as Holium laser enucleation (HoLEP) and Greenlight laser.

In a prospective clinical trial, Mitchell et al. evaluated 33 men with DU, 14 men with detrusor hypocontractility and 19 patients with detrusor acontractility undergoing HoLEP [13]. Impaired bladder contractility was defined using the bladder contractility index (BCI) <100. Pre-operatively each patient underwent an urodynamic assessment. Overall there was a significant reduction in IPSS scores 6-month postoperatively compared to baseline (21.5 vs. 3, $p=0.014$) [13]. Furthermore, Qmax significantly improved (10 vs. 21 mL/s, $p=0.001$), while PVR was significantly reduced (250 vs. 53 mL, $p=0.007$) [13]. In terms of patient satisfaction, 55.6 % of men with

DU were "delighted" with the results [13]. A major limitation of the study was the lack of long-term follow-up data to assess the durability of the treatment response.

Photoselective vaporization (PVP) with the Greenlight laser is a minimally invasive procedure using 532 nm high-powered laser light to ablate obstructing prostatic tissue. Several studies have demonstrated the relative efficiency when treating DU. Monoski et al. retrospectively reviewed 40 men to determine whether preoperative urodynamic parameters can predict outcome in men with urinary retention undergoing PVP [14]. The purpose of the urodynamic study was to identify men with either impaired detrusor contractility (IDC) or detrusor overactivity (DO). IDC was defined using criteria defined by the International Continence Society ref. In total, 8 men had IDC, while 30 had DO pre-operatively. Subjects were followed post-operatively for 12 months. IPSS for men with IDC showed a 25 % reduction from baseline to 12-months (12.0 vs. 9.0) [14]. Furthermore, Qmax showed a 155 % improvement at 12-months post-operatively (4.8 vs 12.3 mL/s) [14]. Lastly, an 80 % reduction was seen in patients' PVR (918.3 vs. 181.5 mL) [14]. Monoski and colleagues noted that men without IDC or DO showed the greatest improvement.

In a study by Cho et al., the impact of HoLEP or PVP on DU was investigated. In the study, Du was defined as a patient having a bladder contractility index of <100. One thousand four-hundred and twenty-three men were recruited and categorized into four different groups: 239 men without DU and 432 with DU were randomized to receive HoLEP treatment. Furthermore, 329 men without DU and 423 men with DU were randomized to receive PVP as a treatment [15]. When comparing patients with and without DU preoperatively, IPSS, subtotal voiding symptom score and Qmax were worse in the DU group [15]. When comparing across procedures, those with DU in the HoLEP groups showed the greatest degree of post-operative improvement in total IPSS, Qmax and subtotal voiding symptom score [15]. However, none of these parameters showed statistical significance. Although this treatment showed relatively good efficacy, researchers concluded that patients with DU seemed to improve to a lesser extent when undergoing PVP or HoLEP compared to those without DU.

These studies suggest that HoLEP and PVP are viable outlet reduction surgeries in patients with DU. The severity of DU can affect surgical efficacy although it has not well defined in these studies. We can speculate that the substantial recovery of spontaneous urination and restoration of some contractility of detrusor muscle is due to the degree of DU being mild, relief of stressed detrusor muscle and minimal damage from operation [13]. By contrast where there is a lack of surgical efficacy there is likely to be a greater degree of impairment of detriusor activity preoperatively. As such, further studies evaluating the differences in impairment of detrusor activity may be beneficial in understanding the variability of surgical outcomes.

Outlet Reduction Surgery for Women

DU is even less well characterized in women than in men and shows a lower prevalence [6]. Choi et al. performed a multi-center study to investigate the prevalence and characteristics of voiding dysfunctions in women across nine hospitals [8].

Seven-hundred and ninety-two women visited clinics with symptoms of lower urinary tract symptoms (LUTS). In order to examine urinary function, researchers performed uroflowmetry and residual urine volume by urethral catherization. For the purposes of this study DU was defined as "Qmax <15 ml/s and detrusor pressure <20 cmH_2O at Qmax" [8]. Of those with voiding difficulty, a total of 13 (12.7 %) of patients had DU. When comparing characteristics of female voiding difficulty, researchers found no significant differences between those with functional BOO or DU, except when looking at detrusor pressure at Qmax BOO = 45.4 ± 18.7 cmH_2O vs. DU = 13.0 ± 4.9 cmH_2O, $P < 0.05$.

Bladder Neck Incisions

For women with BOO at the bladder neck, transurethral bladder-neck incisions (TUI-BN) have been utilized to reduce outlet resistance [16]. The procedure has demonstrated long-term efficacy in restoring spontaneous voiding and relieving voiding difficulties [16]. It is postulated that this procedure may be effective in treating patients, especially women with DU due to potential bladder neck obstruction [16].

In a retrospective study, Jhang et al. 31 assessed female patients with DU who had underwent TUI-BN. The technique was performed using a resectoscope and a diathermy electrode. Incisions were made 5 o'clock and 7 o'clock positions of the bladder neck. Urodynamic parameters were collected for each patient preoperatively to determine any additional etiologies in relation to their DU diagnosis [16]. Three-months post-operatively patients showed a statistically significant improvement in voided volume, Qmax, PVR and voiding efficiency. In total, PVR decreased by 56.3 % when comparing patients post TUI-BN to baseline (391.5 vs 171.1, $p < 0.0001$). Similarly, voiding efficiency, defined as the voided volume/total bladder capacity × 100 %, increased from 5 to 52 %, $p < 0.0001$ [16]. Qmax and voiding volume showed significant improvement amongst this cohort of patients, increasing from 1.10 vs 7.82 mL/s and 22.0 vs 171.9 mL, respectively with a p value <0.0001 [16]. Researchers conclude TUI-BN to be an effective treatment for female patients with DU and bladder neck obstruction given its ability to improve PVR, voiding volume and efficiency and Qmax.

In a long-term follow up study, Jhang et al. again evaluated the effect TUI-BN for female patients with DU. Fifty women who had not responded favorably to other treatment options for DU underwent TUI-BN [17]. At baseline and at each follow-up time point (mean follow-up 61.8 months), urodynamic parameters were obtained. Similarly to their previous study, voiding efficiency (0.0 vs 50 %, $p < 0.0001$), voided volume (0.0 vs 167 mL, $p < 0.0001$), PVR (400 vs 150 mL, $p < 0.0001$) and Qmax (0.0 vs 5.0 mL/s, $p < 0.0001$) all demonstrated significant improvements [17]. Interestingly, maximum detrusor pressure at Qmax (pdetQmax) showed statistically significant improvement as well (0.0 vs 7.5 cmH_2O, $p = 0.002$) [17]. Twenty-six patients reported overall satisfaction following treatment. It is noteworthy "higher Pves compared to a lower Pves was predictive of satisfactory surgical outcomes" [17]. Overall, TUI-BN is an effective treatment for female patients with DU and has shown durable results during the post-operative years (>5 years). However it should be noted that there are a limited number of studies and a lack of randomized-control trials addressing the efficacy of treatment options appropriate for women with DU.

Although limited in the number of studies, TUI-BN may potentially be a treatment option for women with DU who have not responded well to other options. A major shortcoming however in these studies was researchers failed to take into account the clinical severity of the participants' DU. Thus, more research is necessary to determine if TUI-BN can be a safe procedure to alleviate urine retention and other LUTS for women regardless of DU. Furthermore TUI-BN in women comes with attendant risks of stress urinary incontinence and bladder neck contracture and cannot be advocated as a standard approach in clinical practice before more robust data is available as to the safety and efficacy of the technique.

Outlet Reduction Follow-Up

Post-treatment follow-up typically comprises of uroflowmetry, PVR and validated symptom scores such as IPSS. However, more detailed urodynamics such as the pressure flow studies in the bladder are not routinely conducted. As a result, many long-term studies [9, 10] do not have urodynamic data on patients to analyze parameters of improvement. For example, Masumori et al. reported at least 1/3 of the surviving participants were lost to follow up suggesting long-term studies may be subject to bias.

In order to increase the flow and empty the bladder, patients can apply several different physical/behavioral techniques in addition to surgical therapy. Physicians can teach patients to void via the Valsalva maneuver. Also known as Crede voiding, the Valsalva technique involves squeezing the abdominal muscles or application of pressure to the abdomen during urination with voluntary relaxation of the external sphincter [18]. This can help to apply the additional pressure to the weakened bladder to empty. This learned voiding process can be supplemented/guided with pelvic floor therapy training or biofeedback.

Conclusion

DU is a complex condition, with common symptoms overlapping with other bladder disorders. This has likely lead to an underestimation of the incidence of DU within the population [19]. The treatment options in DU are limited in their scope in comparison to those available for patients with overactive bladder. The results from the available studies discussed in this chapter demonstrate that success of outlet reduction is limited and there is risk of adverse effects such as incontinence which is particularly of concern in women. Furthermore, there is a lack of validated methods to determine patient satisfaction after outlet reducing therapies. There is a pressing need for better methods to select those patients most likely to benefit from invasive outlet reducing treatment.

References

1. Chapple CR, Osman NI, Birder L, et al. The underactive bladder: a new clinical concept? Eur Urol. 2015;68(3):351 3.
2. Osman NI, Chapple CR, Abrams P, et al. Detrusor underactivity and the underactive bladder: a new clinical entity? A review of current terminology, definitions, epidemiology, aetiology, and diagnosis. Eur Urol. 2014;65(2):389–98.
3. Oelke M, Rademakers KL, van Koeveringe GA. Unravelling detrusor underactivity: development of a bladder outlet resistance-bladder contractility nomogram for adult male patients with lower urinary tract symptoms. Neurourol Urodyn. 2015. doi: 10.1002/nau.22841
4. Jeong SJ, Kim HJ, Lee YJ, et al. Prevalence and clinical features of detrusor underactivity among elderly with lower urinary tract symptoms: a comparison between men and women. Korean J Urol. 2012;53(5):342–8.
5. Rademakers KL, van Koeveringe GA, Oelke M. Detrusor underactivity in men with lower urinary tract symptoms/benign prostatic obstruction: characterization and potential impact on indications for surgical treatment of the prostate. Curr Opin Urol. 2016;26(1):3–10.
6. Nitti VW. Pressure flow urodynamic studies: the gold standard for diagnosing bladder outlet obstruction. Rev Urol. 2005;7 Suppl 6:S14–21.
7. Winters JC, Dmochowski RR, Goldman HB, et al. Urodynamic studies in adults: AUA/SUFU guideline. J Urol. 2012;188(6 Suppl):2464–72.
8. Choi YS, Kim JC, Lee KS, et al. Analysis of female voiding dysfunction: a prospective, multicenter study. Int Urol Nephrol. 2013;45(4):989–94.
9. Masumori N, Furuya R, Tanaka Y, Furuya S, Ogura H, Tsukamoto T. The 12-year symptomatic outcome of transurethral resection of the prostate for patients with lower urinary tract symptoms suggestive of benign prostatic obstruction compared to the urodynamic findings before surgery. BJU Int. 2010;105(10):1429–33.
10. Tanaka Y, Masumori N, Itoh N, Furuya S, Ogura H, Tsukamoto T. Is the short-term outcome of transurethral resection of the prostate affected by preoperative degree of bladder outlet obstruction, status of detrusor contractility or detrusor overactivity? Int J Urol. 2006;13(11): 1398–404.
11. Thomas AW, Cannon A, Bartlett E, Ellis-Jones J, Abrams P. The natural history of lower urinary tract dysfunction in men: the influence of detrusor underactivity on the outcome after transurethral resection of the prostate with a minimum 10-year urodynamic follow-up. BJU Int. 2004;93(6):745–50.
12. Hsu YC, Lin YH, Chou CY, et al. Economic evaluation study (cheer compliant) laser prostatectomy for benign prostatic hyperplasia: outcomes and cost-effectiveness. Med (Baltimore). 2016;95(5):e2644.
13. Mitchell CR, Mynderse LA, Lightner DJ, Husmann DA, Krambeck AE. Efficacy of holmium laser enucleation of the prostate in patients with non-neurogenic impaired bladder contractility: results of a prospective trial. Urology. 2014;83(2):428–32.
14. Monoski MA, Gonzalez RR, Sandhu JS, Reddy B, Te AE. Urodynamic predictors of outcomes with photoselective laser vaporization prostatectomy in patients with benign prostatic hyperplasia and preoperative retention. Urology. 2006;68(2):312–7.
15. Cho MC, Ha SB, Park J, et al. Impact of detrusor underactivity on surgical outcomes of laser prostatectomy: comparison in serial 12-month follow-up outcomes between potassium-titanyl-

phosphate Photoselective Vaporization of the Prostate (PVP) and Holmium Laser Enucleation of the Prostate (HoLEP). Urology. 2016;91:158–66.
16. Jhang JF, Jiang YH, Lee CL, Kuo HC. Long-term follow up and predictive factors for successful outcome of transurethral incision of the bladder neck in women with detrusor underactivity. J Formos Med Assoc. 2016;115(9):807–13. doi: 10.1016/j.jfma.2015.08.009. Epub 2015 Sep 12.
17. Anderson BB, Pariser JJ, Pearce SM, Volsky J, Bales GT, Chung DE. Safety and Efficacy of Retropubic Mid-Urethral Sling Placement in Women Who Void with Valsalva. Urology. 2016;91:52–7.
18. Bump RC, Mattiasson A, Bo K, et al. The standardization of terminology of female pelvic organ prolapse and pelvic floor dysfunction. Am J Obstet Gynecol. 1996;175(1):10–7.
19. Hoag N, Gani J. Underactive bladder: clinical features, urodynamic parameters, and treatment. Int Neurourol J. 2015;19(3):185–9.

Neurostimulation and Neuromodulation for the Treatment for the Underactive Bladder

8

J. Drossaerts, R. Jairam, G.A. van Koeveringe, and P.E.V. van Kerrebroeck

Key Points

- Several electrical stimulation techniques are available for the treatment of DU.
- The anterior sacral root stimulator is an option to restore volitional voiding in patients with complete spinal cord injury but requires sufficient bladder contractility.
- Sacral neuromodulation has established efficacy in patients with urinary retention but also requires sufficient contractility.
- Transurethral electrotherapy is a promising less invasive option, but randomised studies are required to establish efficacy.

Introduction

According to the ICS detrusor underactivity (DU) can be defined as a decreased strength or duration of detrusor contraction, preventing the timely and efficient emptying of the bladder [1]. The symptom complex of underactive bladder (UAB) has not been formally defined but is characterised by urinary symptoms including hesitancy, straining and incomplete bladder emptying in the absence of an anatomical obstruction.

There are three possible mechanisms by which the UAB can develop [2–4]. Patients in whom the main cause is thought to be an age-related decrease in detrusor

J. Drossaerts, MD • R. Jairam, MD • G.A. van Koeveringe, MD, PhD
P.E.V. Van Kerrebroeck, MD, PhD, MMSc (✉)
Department of Urology, Maastricht University Medical Center+,
PO BOX 5800, Maastricht NL – 6202 AZ, The Netherlands
e-mail: g.van.koeveringe@mumc.nl; p.vankerrebroeck@mumc.nl

C.R. Chapple et al. (eds.), *Underactive Bladder*,
DOI 10.1007/978-3-319-43087-4_8

contractility can be labelled as having idiopathic UAB. It is hypothesised that this process has two phases where a decrease in detrusor strength is preceded by reduced detrusor contraction velocity [5]. The myogenic hypothesis is based on impairment of the bladder smooth muscle function due to an altered excitation-contraction coupling mechanism of the detrusor muscle cells and results in reduced intrinsic myogenic activity of the detrusor. In the neurogenic hypothesis UAB may result from changes in the efferent limb of the micturition reflex, the afferent signals initiating the reflex and the integrative control [4]. Since detrusor contraction and strength are a result of efferent nerve activity which is dependent on sensory input, impaired sensory function can also cause UAB.

Patient with UAB are at risk for the development of chronic renal failure and urinary tract infections. These patients have to rely on an indwelling bladder catheter or clean intermittent catheterisation. Unfortunately effective oral drugs are lacking. Based on our knowledge on the neurophysiology and due to the development of electrical innovations, neurostimulation and neuromodulation have been clinically adopted in the treatment of UAB.

History of Electrical Bladder Stimulation

The first electrical stimulation of the nerve, which resulted in muscle contraction was discovered by Galvani in 1786. After this, [6] was the first who experimented with transected spinal cords in dogs, and our interest in and understanding of basic neurophysiology of micturition began to develop. This led to observations of bladder function in the setting of selective rhizotomy of the pelvic and hypogastric nerves. Also direct stimulation of the bladder through both transurethral and direct detrusor routes was discovered by Saxtorph in 1878. Stimulation of the pelvic nerve and pelvic floor muscle was not well studied until [7] stimulated the pelvic nerve and observed both detrusor muscle and urethral sphincter contractions in a cat.

In 1972 Brindley performed a sacral rhizotomy in paraplegic patients with urine incontinence, and stimulated the anterior branches of the sacral nerves to provoke bladder contraction. After this, Tanagho and co-workers stimulated the sacral root in paraplegic dog with a spiral electrode. They discovered that stimulating the sacral roots resulted in modulation of the external sphincter which in turn inhibited detrusor activity. All of these experiments have led to concepts which are still applicable in the neurostimulation and neuromodulation techniques to date.

Electrical Stimulation of the Underactive Bladder

Neurophysiology

There are two important reflexes which play a role in the bladder storage. The guarding reflex promotes continence and allows contraction of the urinary sphincter during periods of stress [8]. The second reflex is the bladder afferent loop reflex which works through sacral interneurons and activate storage through the pudendal nerve which contract the urethral sphincter. Suprapontine input from the brains can switch these reflexes off to promote voiding.

Pain, pressure, fullness or stretch elicits bladder efferent activity through Aδ or C fibres, and synapse with both parasympathetic efferents (bladder-bladder reflex) and parasympathetic urethral efferents (bladder-urethral reflex). The sensing of a full bladder activates the bladder-bladder reflex which results in contraction of the bladder and leads to a complete emptying. The bladder-urethral reflex induces the smooth muscle of the urethra to relax and the urethral outlet to open reflexively just before the onset of a bladder contraction.

Techniques

Different techniques to promote bladder emptying have evolved through the years.

Nerve Root Stimulation

To activate the micturition centre, spinal cord stimulation was applied. Direct spinal cord stimulation initiates voiding, but the simultaneous urethral sphincter activity prevented proper emptying of the bladder. In 1972 Brindley started sacral root stimulation in combination with rhizotomies of S2, S3 and S4. In this procedure a dorsal sacral rhizotomy is performed in order to eliminate simultaneously bladder and striated sphincter stimulation. Electrodes are placed intradurally to the S2, S3 and S4 nerve roots. The Brindley technique of neurostimulation can be performed in patients with inefficient or non-reflex micturition after spinal cord injury. The principle of the Brindley method relies on post-stimulation voiding, where voiding is prevented during stimulation-induced bladder contractions. Voiding is achieved since the relaxation time of the urethral sphincter is shorter than the relaxation of the detrusor muscle. These prolonged bladder contractions after stimulation result in post stimulus (intermittent) voiding.

Transurethral Electrical Bladder Stimulation

Transurethral electrical bladder stimulation is another method to facilitate bladder emptying. It is hypothesized to activate specific mechanoreceptors in the bladder wall, which activate the intramural motor system, which results in small local muscle contractions. These contractions lead to stimuli which travel through afferent pathways to the corresponding cerebral structures with the occurrence of sensation. These impulses will be responsible for reinforcement of efferent pathways, which cause more coordinated and stronger detrusor contractions. This technique can be performed only in patients with an incomplete spinal cord lesion, with mechanoreceptors still capable of activity, and a detrusor with preserved contractility. Since it also requires a conscious control, an intact cortex is also necessary.

Pudendal Nerve Stimulation

Since the bladder afferent reflex works through the pudendal nerve, this nerve seems to be a logical target for neuromodulation therapies. Stimulation of the nerve may lead to blockage of the urethral sphincter contraction, which leads to relaxation of the sphincter. Peters et al. [9] performed a prospective, single-blinded, randomized crossover trial where 30 patients received either pudendal nerve stimulation or sacral nerve stimulation. Eighty per cent of all patients included had a significant clinical response, and were implanted with an implantable pulse generator. Stimulation of the pudendal nerve resulted in 63 % improvement in symptoms while sacral neuromodulation resulted in 46 % improvement in symptoms.

Sacral Neuromodulation

Sacral neuromodulation is a treatment option in patients with overactive bladder syndrome (OAB) with or without urinary urgency incontinence but also in patients with UAB or non-obstructive urinary retention (NOR), if conservative treatment fails. It was developed by Tanagho and Smith [10], and since then the technique has undergone major developments.

Since it still remains unclear which exact patients will benefit from sacral neuromodulation treatment, the procedure consists of two stages: the first stage where an electrode is placed along the third sacral nerve through the 3rd sacral foramen, and the second stage where the implantable pulse generator is connected to the electrode and implanted subcutaneously. Traditionally, a temporarily lead (unipolar wire electrode) was placed in the sacral foramen S3 and a test stimulation of 4–7 days was performed. Since this lead was not fixed, patients were at high risk for lead migration. Spinelli et al. [11, 12] modified this technique by using a minimally invasive percutaneous approach, which later also included the implantation of a definitive electrode with barbed hooks (a tined lead). Since there was no need for an open procedure but a Seldinger technique could be performed and thus making the use of local anesthesia possible.

Siegel et al. presented long-term results of a multicentre study where 42 patients were implanted and completed 1.5 year of follow-up [13]. Voiding diaries showed a significant reduction in average volume per catheterization. While 70 % reported a 50 % or greater reduction in average volume per catheterization including 58 % who eliminated use of catheterization. A prospective study of Van Kerrebroeck et al. observed a significant decrease of number of catheterizations per day, and a clinical success rate of 58 % 5 years after implantation [14].

Conclusions

Several electrical stimulation techniques are available for the treatment of the underactive bladder. Anterior sacral root stimulation after selective posterior sacral rhizotomy (the Brindley technique) is only possible in selected patients with a complete spinal cord injury and preserved contractility of the detrusor. Sacral neuromodulation is clinically available and FDA approved for patients with an underactive bladder, that react well during trial stimulation. Long-term results are available and seem persistent. In patients were sacral neuromodulation fails or yields insufficient result, pudendal nerve stimulation is an (experimental) alternative.

Literature

1. Abrams P, Cardozo L, Fall M, Griffiths D, Rosier P, Ulmsten U, et al. The standardisation of terminology of lower urinary tract function: report from the Standardisation Sub-committee of the International Continence Society. NeurourolUrodyn. 2002;21(2):167–78.
2. Tyagi P, Smith PP, Kuchel GA, de Groat WC, Birder LA, Chermansky CJ, et al. Pathophysiology and animal modeling of underactive bladder. Int Urol Nephrol. 2014;46 Suppl 1:S11–21.
3. Li X, Liao L. Updates of underactive bladder: a review of the recent literature. Int Urol Nephrol. 2016;48(6):919–30.
4. van Koeveringe GA, Vahabi B, Andersson KE, Kirschner-Hermans R, Oelke M. Detrusor underactivity: a plea for new approaches to a common bladder dysfunction. NeurourolUrodyn. 2011;30(5):723–8.
5. Cucchi A, Quaglini S, Guarnaschelli C, Rovereto B. Urodynamic findings suggesting two-stage development of idiopathic detrusor underactivity in adult men. Urology. 2007;70(1):75–9.
6. Magendie F. Expériences sur les fonctions des racines des nerfs rachidiens. Journal de physiologie expérimentale et de pathologie, 1822;2:276–279.
7. Dees JE. Contraction of the urinary bladder produced by electric stimulation. Preliminary report. Invest Urol 1965;15:539–547.
8. Leng WW, Chancellor MB. How sacral nerve stimulation neuromodulation works. Urol Clin North Am. 2005;32(1):11–8.
9. Peters KM, Feber KM, Bennett RC. Sacral versus pudendal nerve stimulation for voiding dysfunction: a prospective, single-blinded, randomized, crossover trial. NeurourolUrodyn. 2005;24(7):643–7.
10. Tanagho EA, Schmidt RA. Bladder pacemaker: scientific basis and clinical future. Urology. 1982;20(6):614–9.
11. Spinelli M, Giardiello G, Arduini A, van den Hombergh U. New percutaneous technique of sacral nerve stimulation has high initial success rate: preliminary results. Eur Urol. 2003;43(1):70–4.
12. Spinelli M, Giardiello G, Gerber M, Arduini A, van den Hombergh U, Malaguti S. New sacral neuromodulation lead for percutaneous implantation using local anesthesia: description and first experience. J Urol. 2003;170(5):1905–7.
13. Siegel S, Noblett K, Mangel J, Griebling TL, Sutherland SE, Bird ET, et al. Results of a prospective, randomized, multicenter study evaluating sacral neuromodulation with InterStim therapy compared to standard medical therapy at 6-months in subjects with mild symptoms of overactive bladder. NeurourolUrodyn. 2015;34:224–30.
14. van Kerrebroeck PE, van Voskuilen AC, Heesakkers JP, Lycklama a Nijholt AA, Siegel S, Jonas U, et al. Results of sacral neuromodulation therapy for urinary voiding dysfunction: outcomes of a prospective, worldwide clinical study. J Urol. 2007;178:2029–34.

Reduction Cystoplasty

9

A. Kavanagh, J. Stewart, and T. Boone

Key Points

- Reduction cystoplasty is a surgical intervention aimed at reducing bladder capacity to a 'normal' range.
- Within the limitations of retrospective case series with mixed pathology and varied surgical approach, patients with acontractile bladders tend to do more poorly than those with hypocontractile detrusor function.
- Long term studies fail to demonstrate a sustained benefit and suggest reduction cystoplasty has limited long term effects on bladder volume
- Overall, reduction cystoplasty has not been definitively proven to yield long-term success in most patients and its use remains debatable

Defining large bladder capacity (LBC) is difficult as considerable variation in bladder capacity exists even among healthy young adults [1]. Despite a large storage potential, some individuals are able to generate a sufficient bladder contraction to drain the bladder with an appropriate post-void residual and avoid unwanted sequelae. In a recent review of 100 subjects with LBC (range: 700 ml – 5.0 L), the primary pathophysiologic diagnoses were bladder outlet obstruction in 48 % of cases Detrusor underactivity (DU) in 11 %, absent detrusor contractility in 24 % and normal detrusor pressure uroflow study in 17 % [2]. DU is characterized by a low amplitude detrusor contraction and synchronous low uroflow (Qmax) and/or detrusor contraction of insufficient duration to empty the bladder at a normal flow

A. Kavanagh, MD (✉)
Department of Urologic Sciences, University of British Columbia, Vancouver, BC, Canada

J. Stewart, MD • T. Boone, MD, PhD (✉)
Department of Urology, Houston Methodist Hospital, Houston, TX, USA
e-mail: TBoone3@houstonmethodist.org

C.R. Chapple et al. (eds.), *Underactive Bladder*,
DOI 10.1007/978-3-319-43087-4_9

rate [3]. In the setting of LBC with DU, myogenic decompensation of the bladder with excessive urinary capacity and chronic urinary retention is a common clinical scenario [4].

When LBC is accompanied by lower urinary tract symptoms it is important to determine detrusor function, as corrective outlet surgery may fail to address elevated residual volume in the setting of DU. Some authors advocate addressing LBC with reduction cystoplasty, a surgical intervention aimed at reducing bladder capacity to a 'normal' range.

Although removing bladder tissue to improve functional outcomes seems counterintuitive, the premise can be explained in relation to Laplace's law. This law states that P = k*T/R, where P is the cavitary pressure, k is a constant, T is the wall tension, and R is the radius of the chamber. Assuming wall tension remains constant, intraluminal voiding pressure should increase by 25 % if the volume is decreased by half [5]. Similar initiatives to treat dilated cardiomyopathy have investigated reduction of the left ventricular diameter in patients with heart failure to improve left ventricular ejection fraction. Studies in this setting have demonstrated improved functional outcomes despite high acute morbidity and a significant failure rate [6].

The first documented attempt at surgical correction of LBC using reduction cystoplasty was performed in 1937 with reported improvements in obstructive symptoms, a decrease in the frequency of urinary tract infections and a permanent reduction in the volume of residual urine [7]. **Subsequent documented evidence of the therapeutic benefit of this procedure is scant with numerous small case series with variable pathology, diverse surgical approaches to both the bladder and outlet and with very limited follow-up** [5, 8–11].

Commonly employed techniques of reduction cystoplasty include transection and resection of the superior bladder dome (Klarskov et al. [8]), **vesicoplication** (Stewart et al. [9]) **and detrusor wrap** (Zoedler et al. [12]). The Stewart method involves a series of invagination sutures along the circumference of the bladder, converting the vault into a piston force for evacuating the urine. In the Zoedler technique (Fig. 9.1) the front and the back wall of the bladder are incised down to the trigonal area. In one hemisphere the mucosa is removed, and from the other hemisphere the extravesical fat is cut away. The two parts are then passed over each other so that the detrusor layers are close to each other. As no muscle tissue is resected, the result is a detrusor of double thickness [12].

Kinn et al. [11] retrospectively reviewed 10 patients of mixed pathology who were randomly assigned to either the Zoedler or Stewart reduction cystoplasty and were then followed for a mean of 25 months. Male patients were treated with concomitant radical incision of the bladder neck and females were treated with aggressive urethral dilation. After reduction cystoplasty, bladder capacity and residual volume were significantly decreased. Urodynamic assessment after the procedure revealed no significant improvement in urinary flow rate or detrusor contractility compared to pre-operative evaluation. Functional outcomes of urinary tract infection were improved through the course of follow-up, but it remains unclear if this is related to the bladder outlet procedure or the reduction cystoplasty [11]. Similar

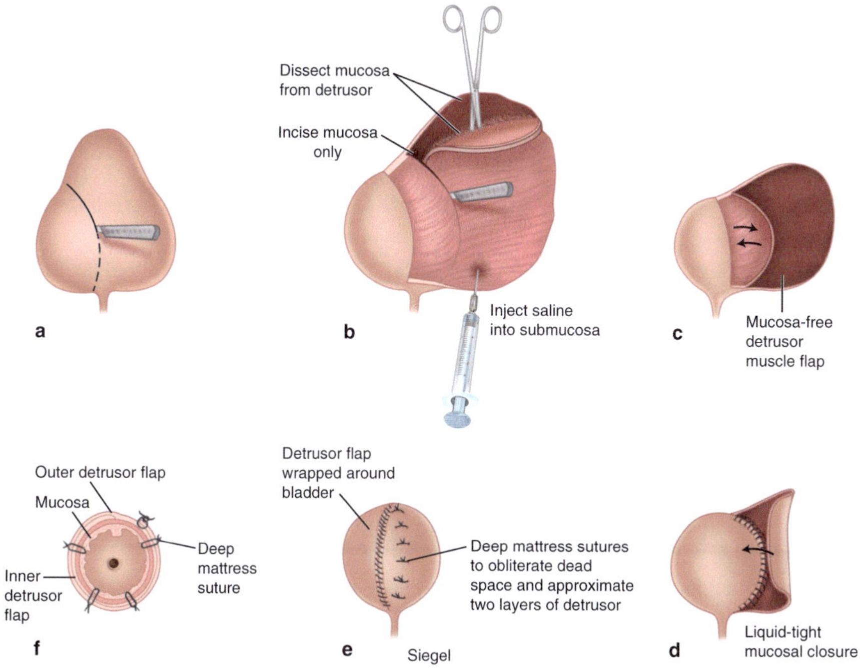

Fig. 9.1 Zoedler detrusor wrap technique of reduction cystoplasty. (**a**) Bladder incision, (**b**) Dissection of mucosal flap from detrusor, (**c**) Mobilization of detrusor flap, (**d**, **e**) Mucosal opposition with volume reduction, (**f**) Out detrusor flap secured in 'vest over pants' fashion (Figure provided by Hanna et al. [10])

findings were obtained by Klarskov et al. [8] in a group of 11 patients of mixed pathology treated with resection of the bladder dome with a median follow-up of 4 years. Recently, Thorner et al. [13] published a retrospective review of 8 patients with mixed pathology in the setting of impaired detrusor contractility and elevated post-void residual greater than 600 ml. At 1 year following reduction cystoplasty, significant improvements in residual urine were observed, with only one patient requiring self-catheterization.

One of the largest series of patients with common pathology evaluated 21 diabetic patients treated with cystoenteric conversion of their pancreas transplantation and concomitant reduction cystoplasty. The primary pathology of subjects was diabetic cystopathy with failure to empty. With a follow-up of 2.5 years after reduction cystoplasty, mean bladder capacity decreased from 650 to 362 ml according to urodynamic testing ($p < 0.0001$). Post-void residual urine volume decreased from 330 to 79 ml ($p < 0.07$) and voiding efficiency increased from 53 to 77 % ($p < 0.10$) [14].

One of the longest term follow-up studies of reduction cystoplasty patients was published by Bukowski and Perlmutter in 1994 [5]. A cohort of 11 boys with severe prune belly syndrome including megacystis manifestation underwent genitourinary reconstruction. Reduction cystoplasty was undertaken as part of a comprehensive reconstruction in an attempt to improve bladder emptying and decrease the risk of infection and possible deterioration of renal function. The bladder dome and urachal remnant were removed in an attempt to minimize diverticula and reapproximate a more spherical shape. After removing the bladder dome, a fusiform strip of mucosa was excised from one side and a 3-layer 'vest over pants' closure was performed corresponding to the Zoedler technique (Fig. 9.1). Average initial reduction in bladder volume was 52 % in the 9 patients with available follow-up. After 7.7 years of follow-up (range 1.5–14) bladder volumes corrected for age were essentially unchanged or greater than corrected preoperative volumes. The investigators concluded reduction cystoplasty had limited long-term effect on bladder volume [5].

In addition to questionable short and long term outcomes, some authors have suggested that the process of reduction cystoplasty may cause conversion of a low pressure, compliant bladder to a high pressure, noncompliant organ, thereby placing the upper urinary tracts at risk [15]. Whether this remains a function of short-term follow-up or an insignificant concern remains debatable. However, the longest term studies available fail to demonstrate either significant reflux or development of hydronephrosis [5].

In conclusion, reduction cystoplasty seems to be an attractive alternative for patients with chronic urinary retention and a large decompensated bladder. However, results proving efficacy are lacking. **Like many reconstructive procedures performed in the past to make the anatomy look better, the actual physiological outcomes have not paralleled the surgery.** Within the limitations of retrospective case series with mixed pathology and varied surgical approach, patients with acontractile bladders tend to do more poorly than those with hypocontractile detrusor function [8, 10]**. Long term studies fail to demonstrate a sustained benefit and suggest reduction cystoplasty has limited long term effects on bladder volume** [5]**. Overall, reduction cystoplasty has not been definitively proven to yield long-term success in most patients and its use remains debatable.**

References

1. Wyndaele JJ. Normality in urodynamics studied in healthy adults. J Urol. 1999;161(3): 899–902.
2. Purohit RS, Blaivas JG, Saleem KL, Sandhu J, Weiss JP, Reddy B, et al. The pathophysiology of large capacity bladder. J Urol. 2008;179(3):1006–11.
3. Blaivas JG, Groutz A. Bladder outlet obstruction nomogram for women with lower urinary tract symptomatology. NeurourolUrodyn. 2000;19(5):553–64.
4. Weir J, Jaques PF. Large-capacity bladder. A urodynamic survey. Urology. 1974;4(5):544–8.
5. Bukowski TP, Perlmutter AD. Reduction cystoplasty in the prune belly syndrome: a long-term followup. J Urol. 1994;152(6 Pt 1):2113–6.
6. Batista RJ, Verde J, Nery P, Bocchino L, Takeshita N, Bhayana JN, et al. Partial left ventriculectomy to treat end-stage heart disease. Ann Thorac Surg. 1997;64(3):634–8.
7. Lm O. Management of atonic bladder due to obstruction of vesical neck. Southern Med J. 1937;30(1):519–24.

8. Klarskov P, Holm-Bentzen M, Larsen S, Gerstenberg T, Hald T. Partial cystectomy for the myogenic decompensated bladder with excessive residual urine. Urodynamics, histology and 2–13 years follow-up. Scand J Urol Nephrol. 1988;22(4):251–6.
9. Stewart HH. The surgical treatment of severe chronic retention without large diverticula. Br J Urol. 1966;38(6):685–95.
10. Hanna MK. New concept in bladder remodeling. Urology. 1982;19(1):6–12.
11. Kinn AC. The lazy bladder–appraisal of surgical reduction. Scand J Urol Nephrol. 1985;19(2):93–9.
12. Zoedler D. Zur operativen Behandlung der Blasenatonie. Z Urol. 1964;19(1):743.
13. Thorner DA, Blaivas JG, Tsui JF, Kashan MY, Weinberger JM, Weiss JP. Outcomes of reduction cystoplasty in men with impaired detrusor contractility. Urology. 2014;83(4):882–6.
14. Black PC, Plaskon LA, Miller J, Bakthavatsalam R, Kuhr CS, Marsh CL. Cystoenteric conversion and reduction cystoplasty for treatment of bladder dysfunction after pancreas transplantation. J Urol. 2003;170(5):1913–7.
15. Kinahan TJ, Churchill BM, McLorie GA, Gilmour RF, Khoury AE. The efficiency of bladder emptying in the prune belly syndrome. J Urol. 1992;148(2 Pt 2):600–3.

Therapeutic Approaches, to Restore or Augment Detrusor Contractility "Bladder Wrap Procedures"

10

Gommert A. van Koeveringe and Kevin L.J. Rademakers

Key Points

- Several clinical reports on bladder wrap procedures to augment bladder contractility are described in the literature.
- Rectus abdominis and rectus femoris wraps have not shown evidence of clinical efficacy.
- Latissmus dorsi detrusor myoplasty is the most studied technique with modest mid term results.
- Bladder wraps represent major surgery and should be considered experimental until more evidence is available confirming its efficacy; it is likely to be of most benefit to younger motivated patients who wish to avoid intermittent self-cathetrisation.

Several non pharmacological options to augment bladder contractility have been attempted through the years. For the most part these options have been unsuccessful except in very specific situations. The option to stimulate the muscle electrically was found to be feasible in patients with unexplained retention but has major limitations such as issues with battery life and implant infection or failure. Surgical procedures for incomplete or inefficient emptying of the bladder such as reduction cystoplasty have been reported, which do not actually augment the contractility of

G.A. van Koeveringe, MD, PhD (✉)
Professor and Chairman, Departmentof Urology,
Maastricht University Medical Center+, Maastricht, The Netherlands
e-mail: g.van.koeveringe@mumc.nl

K.L.J. Rademakers
Maastricht University Medical Centre, Maastricht, The Netherlands
e-mail: kevin.rademakers@mumc.nl

C.R. Chapple et al. (eds.), *Underactive Bladder*,
DOI 10.1007/978-3-319-43087-4_10

the bladder but merely decrease the compliance of the bladder and can put the functional contractile range of bladder filling at a lower level. There are only very few circumstances where this is recommended and moreover there is a significant risk of creating a high-pressure system leading to kidney damage and sometimes overflow incontinence.

One of the first reports of a bladder wrap procedure for an a-contractile detrusor was by Messing and coworkers in 1985 [1]. The authors described a surgical procedure on a patient with Prune Belly Syndrome. From two sides a pedicled flap of the rectus femoris muscle was detached at the knee and sutured to the bladder dome. Voiding afterwards was described as follows: "At no time has he consciously flexed the hips and/or extended the knees to void". This technique was not repeated on a larger series. In 1990, Zhang and colleagues described an enveloping procedure of the bladder with a flap of the rectus abdominis muscle for the treatment of a patient with a neurogenic bladder [2]. The procedure was performed in 18 patients but the functional results were not satisfactory due to the fact that the rectus was sutured to the bladder itself most probably evoking a squeeze by stretching movement and not an effective downward movement of the bladder. A major issue in procedures using rectus muscle is the segmental innervation of the muscle which leaves the muscle denervated for the large part after a major dissection. Despite this failure, Chancellor et al. 1994 and Savage et al. 2000 studied innervated rectus abdominis muscle transposition in an animal model and both concluded it was feasible [3, 4], however there have not been any further clinical studies in the literature.

An alternative muscle, that is not segmentally innervated and can be transplanted as a free flap is the Latissimus dorsi muscle. The ability of this latissimus dorsi as a musculocutaneous flap was initially discovered by Tansini in 1906 [5]. However, it was not until 1976 that the latissimus dorsi flap became established in reconstructive surgery, as a muscle flap and a musculocutaneous flap. In 1994 von Heyden *and coworkers* described for the first time the use of the latissimus dorsi muscle to augment bladder contractility as a free-muscle flap in dogs [6]. The transposed latissimus dorsi flap was only able to evacuate urine to less than 50 % of the capacity. In 1998 Stenz*l* and colleagues published their first experience with latissismus dorsi detrusor myoplasty (LDDM) in three patients, followed by a series of publications in more patients with an acontractile bladder [7].

The Latissimus Dorsi Detrusor Myoplasty

In 1997 and 1998, Stenzl and Ninkovic published preliminary reports demonstrating effective functional results in experiments using a "tension-torsion" wrap of the Latissimus dorsi muscle around the bladder in dogs [8, 9]. Later, the same team published functional results in humans using a similar procedure [10–12]. The surgical procedure needs a specialized multidisciplinary team of urologists and plastic reconstructive surgeons with experience in functional reconstruction. The plastic reconstructive surgeons harvest the Latissimus dorsi preferably at the non-dominant arm. At least two thirds of the muscle is used as a free muscle flap. The muscle has one bundle that includes the thoracodorsal nerve for innervation of the whole muscle and the thoracodorsal vessels for the circulation. These structures are dissected and left long enough to enable future microsurgical re-anastomosis. The in-situ length of the muscle is marked with sutures or clips on the inside of the muscle to enable adequate repositioning at a functional muscle length.

Through a Pfannenstiel incision, the urologist exposes the dome of the bladder via a retroperitoneal approach. Deep in the pelvis the sacro-ischio-spinal ligaments are identified for deep latissimus dorsi muscle attachment. The dorsal attachment is done on a vicryl mesh pulled alongside the bladder neck and attached anteriorly to coopers ligament in the male and to the vaginal vault in the female patients. The anterior part of the muscle is attached to the caudal anterior pelvic ring that involves the pubic bone.

The latissimus dorsi muscle is positioned upside down on the bladder dome and attached to the structures indicated above. For the neurovascular anastomosis, the lowest branches of the intercostal nerve (innervating the rectus abdominis muscle) and the ipsilateral inferior epigastric vein and artery are identified. Then a microscopic end-to-end coaptation of the thoracodorsal nerve to the earlier identified lower branches of the subcostal nerve is performed by the plastic surgeon.

Until recently, there are four studies describing small case series of patients treated with LDDM [7, 10–12]. This is mainly due to, the latissimus dorsi detrusor myoplasty being regarded as an experimental surgical procedure. The mean or median age among the different studies varied from 39 to 42 years, with a postoperative follow-up ranging from 8 to 89 months. Most of the patients carried out CISC before LDDM was performed (17–319 months).

In three of the four published LDDM studies, outcome of the treatment was defined as 'complete', 'partial' or 'no' response, depending on the post void residual (PVR) and amount of CISC. A 'complete' response was defined as spontaneous voiding after LDDM with a post void residual (PVR) of less than 100 ml. The first article of Stenzl *and colleagues* described the first three patients successfully treated with LDDM with a PVR ranging from 0 to 95 ml [7]. Subsequently, the other studies showed a complete response rate varying from 70.8 to 85.0 % [10–12]. The largest of the four studies, a multicenter study discussing the long-term results, showed a success rate after the procedure of 70.8 % (17/24 patients), with a partial response in another 12.5 % (3/24 patients) of the patients. The same study showed absence of UTI's after LDDM in the group of complete responders. However, as in the other studies a specific decrease in frequency in UTI's is not mentioned.

The long-term outcome after LDDM has to be determined still, however the studies mentioned above show promising success rates. These studies had a wide follow-up range, from 8 up 89 months, with a mean follow-up period of 46 months. When comparing this to the relatively young mean age of the included patients, these results most probably reflect short to midterm outcome rather than the long-term outcome. So although the complete response rate in this study looks promising, it still remains to be seen how the LDDM results in this relatively young group of patients are 10 years after surgery.

In two of the articles both the outcome and the initial, preoperative diagnosis were given per patient. In both case series there was a minority of patients with idiopathic bladder acontractility – in five and two patients - respectively. Remarkably the outcome after LDDM in this group was worse compared to the patients with other indications. In the first study two of the five idiopathic acontractile bladder patients were non-responders and another patient was a partial responder, making the complete response rate of the idiopathic group in this study only 40 %. In the second study one of the two patients with an idiopathic acontractile bladder did not manage to void voluntarily and CISC status was unchanged. In general, these idiopathic patients appear to be much older (mostly ≥60 years) than the other patients selected for LDDM. Therefore, it is suggested to use extra caution in this specific group of patients in which no clear origin of bladder acontractility is found. Furthermore, the use additional diagnostic evaluations should be considered in this group. In the somatic area, an ambulatory urodynamic investigation (AUM) is advised and in addition a proper psychological and psychiatric evaluation should be considered.

The complications following a Latissimus dorsi detrusor myoplasty procedure have been described as mild to moderate in the available studies. Also donor side complications were described moderate to low, which is in accordance with other studies on the use of the latissimus dorsi muscle for different indications.

Measurement of Postoperative Improvement of Voiding Function

The primary outcome measurement after a bladder wrap procedure should be, improvement of the voiding and catheterization diary, with improvement of amount of catheterisations per day combined with the volume of each catheterisation. Ideally, pre-and postoperative bladder contractility parameters should be compared in addition in order to evaluate the function of the LDDM. However, all published studies on LDDM use different detrusor contraction parameters, reflecting the continuous search for a reliable parameter to measure bladder contractility during a pressure-flow study.

In general, patients eligible for LDDM show no micturition contraction on preoperative pressure-flow study and most of these patients are even unable to void. As all contractility parameters are flow dependent, it is impossible to evaluate preoperative detrusor contractility in this patient group. Moreover, without the presence of a urinary flow proper definition of the outlet obstruction gradient and sphincter function measurement are also not possible to evaluate. It would be important to evaluate this as postoperative inability to void might be caused by a non-functioning bladder wrap or by high bladder outlet obstruction gradient.

The most recent study on LDDM uses Bladder Contractility Index (BCI) as postoperative contractility measurement [12]. In the BCI formula ($5Q_{max} \times pdetQ_{max}$) detrusor pressure at maximum flow ($pdetQ_{max}$) and maximum flow (Q_{max}) are included [13]. The first problem that arises is that BCI reflects detrusor pressure and not actually detrusor work, as the maximum Watts factor does approximate detrusor work. A post-LDDM measurement of BCI can be acceptable because of increased bladder contractility after LDDM or can be caused by a more effective transmission of the abdominal pressure to the bladder, both resulting in increased urinary flow. A normal BCI after LDDM does not necessarily indicate the presence of bladder contractility/bladder work. Postoperative measurement of the maximum Watts factor (W_{max}) is thought to give better insight in postoperative bladder work and to be less dependent on the obstruction grade compared to BCI [14]. To give a better insight on the ratio of bladder work and bladder outlet obstruction in the postoperative setting, the Maastricht-Hannover nomogram could be applied [15]. In addition, the rate of isovolumetric substracted bladder pressure (t_{20-80}) on a pressure-flow curvature has been suggested recently as detrusor contractility parameter as it is significantly associated with components of bladder contractility, and only weakly correlated to BCI [16]. With the increasing amount of bladder function restoring (surgical) options postoperative contractility measurements should be carried out unambiguously among different studies. This way study results from different studies will be comparable in the future.

Conclusions

In general, the LDDM is an extensive surgical procedure with modest midterm results only to be performed in specialised centres. In addition, the procedure is only reserved for a highly selected group of patients. Therefore, other less invasive and morbid options to reconstruct the bladder muscle represent an upcoming field within (functional) urology and also for this purpose, tissue engineering is gaining interest amongst researchers and clinicians.

References

1. Messing EM, Dibbell DG, Belzer FO. Bilateral rectus femoris pedicle flaps for detrusor augmentation in the prune belly syndrome. J Urol. 1985;134(6):1202–5.
2. Zhang YH, Shao QA, Wang JM. Enveloping the bladder with displacement of flap of the rectus abdominis muscle for the treatment of neurogenic bladder. J Urol. 1990;144(5):1194–5.
3. Michael B, et al. Detrusor-myoplasty, innervated rectus muscle transposition study, and functional effect on the spinal cord injury Rat model. NeurourolUrodyn. 1994;13(5):547–57.
4. Van Savage JG, John G, et al. Electrically stimulated detrusor myoplasty. J Urol. 2000;164(3):969–72.
5. Tansini I. Coverage of the anterior chest wall following mastectomy. Guz Mal Ital. 1906;57:141.
6. Von Heyden B, et al. The latissimus dorsi muscle for detrusor assistance: functional recovery after nerve division and repair. J Urol. 1994;151(4):1081–7.
7. Stenzl A, et al. Restoration of voluntary emptying of the bladder by transplantation of innervated free skeletal muscle. Lancet. 1998;351(9114):1483–5.
8. Stenzl A, et al. Free neurovascular transfer of latissimus dorsi muscle to the bladder. I. Experimental studies. J Urol. 1997;157(3):1103–8.
9. Ninkovic M, et al. Functional urinary bladder wall substitute using a free innervated latissimus dorsi muscle flap. Plastic Reconstructive Surg. 1997;100(2):402–11.

10. Stenzl A. Free neurovascular transfer of latissimus dorsi muscle for the treatment of bladder acontractility: II. clinical results. Int Braz J Urol Off J Braz Soc Urol. 2003;29(2):179–80.
11. Stenzl A, Strasser H, Klima G, et al. Reconstruction of the lower urinary tract using autologous muscle transfer and cell seeding: current status and future perspectives. World J Urol. 2000;18(1):44–50.
12. Gakis G, Ninkovic M, Van Koeveringe GA, et al. Functional detrusor myoplasty for bladder acontractility: long-term results. J Urol. 2011;185(2):593–9.
13. Abrams P. Bladder outlet obstruction index, bladder contractility index and bladder voiding efficiency: three simple indices to define bladder voiding function. BJU Int. 1999;84:14–5.
14. Lecamwasam HS, et al. The maximum watts factor as a measure of detrusor contractility independent of outlet resistance. NeurourolUrodyn. 1998;17(6):621–35.
15. Oelke M, Rademakers KL, Van Koeveringe GA. Unravelling detrusor underactivity: development of a bladder outlet resistance—bladder contractility nomogram for adult male patients with lower urinary tract symptoms. Neurourol Urodyn. 2015 Jul 31. doi: 10.1002/nau.22841. [Epub ahead of print].
16. Fry CH, et al. Estimation of bladder contractility from intravesical pressure–volume measurements. Neurourol Urodyn. 2016 Jun 6. doi: 10.1002/nau.23047. [Epub ahead of print].

Tissue Engineering and Cell Therapy for Underactive Bladder: Current and Future Approaches

11

Reem Aldamanhori, Nadir I. Osman, and Christopher R. Chapple

Key Points

- Tissue engineering of whole bladders for replacement for oncologic purposes or congenital bladder dysfunction replacement has been investigated for over a decade.
- The major challenge with whole bladder engineering is achieving a functional innervation, which has thus far not been possible.
- Stem cell injection therapy into the bladder wall or site of neural injury using adult derived stem cells offers a more practical alternative, however only few small animal studies are available.

Introduction

Regenerative medicine in the form of cell therapy and tissue engineering has been applied clinically in urological practice for over a decade for uses such as grafts in substitution urethroplasty [1] and injection therapy in patients with stress urinary incontinence [2]. *De novo* bladder tissue engineering came to the fore a decade ago with the report of the first clinical study using laboratory grown bladders in the paediatric patients [3]. Although clinical uptake of such technologies has been slow there is growing body of literature evaluating regenerative medicine

R. Aldamanhori (✉)
Department of Urology, University of Dammam, Sheffield, UK
e-mail: reem.baher@gmail.com

N.I. Osman • C.R. Chapple
Department of Urology, Royal Hallamshire Hospital, Sheffield, UK
e-mail: nadirosman@hotmail.com; c.r.chapple@shef.ac.uk

C.R. Chapple et al. (eds.), *Underactive Bladder*,
DOI 10.1007/978-3-319-43087-4_11

approaches for urological diseases in animal models. In this chapter we will discuss the general principles of tissue engineering and stem cell injection therapy as they relate to detrusor underactivity (DU)/underactive bladder (UAB) and available published data.

Basic Principles of Tissue Engineering

Tissue engineering has been defined as "an interdisciplinary field that applies the principles of engineering and life sciences toward the development of biological substitutes that restore, maintain, or improve tissue function or a whole organ"[4]. The approach utilizes biocompatible materials to act as scaffolds for cells. Scaffolds are either composed of natural materials (e.g. porcine small intestinal submucosa) or synthetic polymers (e.g. polyglycolic acid). The cell source can be allogenous but more commonly autologous. The classic approach consists of expanding a population of cells, seeding the cells on the scaffold and culturing the cells on scaffolds, with or without the addition of cytokines and/or growth factors, in the laboratory to develop an engineered tissue substitute. Alternatively tissue inductive scaffolds, which may contain cytokines/growth factors, can be implanted which rely on the ingrowth of cells from the host. Once implanted the aim is for the tissue substitute to remodel into a site-specific functional tissue.

Bladder Tissue Engineering

Much has been published on tissue engineering for bladder substitution or augmented reconstruction in patients with both malignant and benign disease [5]. The main driver for this approach has been to avoid the risk of long-term metabolic complications, urinary stone formation, urinary tract infection, upper tract deterioration and risk of malignancy with the use of small or large intestinal segments in the urinary tract. In addition the lack of volitional contraction of bowel segments which often necessitates drainage using intermittent catheters makes the its use less than ideal as a bladder substitute. For these reasons researchers have attempted to develop bladders using combinations of bioresorbable scaffolds and cells.

Developing a tissue engineered bladder substitute presents major challenges as the bladder is not just a muscular bag with a barrier function but has unique and complex physiological properties, that allow it store urine at low pressure, sense increasing volume and contract in a coordinated to fashion with outlet relaxation to empty effectively when socially appropriate. To fulfill this role, there is a need for intact bladder innervation, central processing of neural signals and functioning detrusor myocytes, notwithstanding the important role the urothelium may play in the micturition reflex.

It is fair to say that attempts thus far to develop a tissue engineered bladder have fallen short in emulating this complex organ. Moreover, no studies have addressed the specific problem of DU/UAB. We will discuss the key practical and theoretical considerations in developing a tissue-engineered bladder as they relate to DU/UAB rather than give detailed exposition of the all studies to date.

The Scaffold

Scaffolds can be derived from decelluarised animal tissue (e.g. porcine small intestinal submucosa), natural polymers (e.g. collagen) or synthetic polymers (e.g. polyglycolic acid). Scaffolds should be porous to permit diffusion of nutrients and cell migration both *in vitro* and *in vivo*. There are general advantages and disadvantages with using each approach and these have been detailed in Table 11.1. For the purpose of bladder tissue engineering a bioresorbable scaffold is preferable over non-degradable materials due to the risk of encrustation and stone formation on contact with urine with the latter. However with bioresporbable materials there is concern with regards to rapid degradation leading to scarring and contracture. Biomechanical properties are important but the key parameters are yet to be defined, intuitively the biomechanical characteristic in keeping with a healthy bladder are desirable. At a very basic level the engineered bladder should have the requisite strength not to rupture during urine storage whilst having a degree of elasticity to avoid problems associated with poor compliance. It is however a much more complex task to develop a scaffold that facilitates the development of a bladder that recreates the properties and arrangement of bladder smooth muscle and its surrounding extracellular matrix, in addition to the sympathetic innervation which is thought to permit receptive relaxation.

The Cells

There is a growing consensus that to large tissue defects or large organs such as the bladder a cellular component to the tissue engineered constructed preferable as reliance of cellular ingrowth to cover large areas is unpredictable [18]. An important question is thus which cell type or types should be used. Clearly the two main cell types that are needed are urothelial and smooth muscle cells. Autologous cells are preferable to avoid the risk of rejection and infectious disease transmission. Urothelial cells can be obtained from bladder biopsies or alternatively protocols have developed to extract urothelial cells from the urine or bladder washes. Alternatively "wet" tissue such as the buccal mucosa could fulfill the barrier function of the bladder but still require a biopsy albeit one which could be taken under a local rather a general anaesthetic as is the case with bladder biopsy. Autologous smooth muscle cells can also be obtained from the native bladder although the wisdom of using such an approach in a patient with a diseased (neuropathic or otherwise) bladder could be questioned. Nevertheless there is evidence that autologous cells from diseased bladder cultured on scaffolds have similar functional performance as those from healthy bladders [18, 19].

Table 11.1 Advantages and disadvantages of different biomaterials for bladder tissue engineering

	Advantage	Disadvantage
Acellular matrix	Biodegradable [6]	Tissue integration not optimal
	Biocompatible	May induce scar tissue (may prevent bladder contraction)
	Although acellular, growth factors are still persevered [7].	Lack f modulation in the healing process [8]
	Do not exhibit any immunogenic rejection [9]	It is challenging to preserve proteins and growth factors with decellularization techniques [8]
	Wider variation in composition and physical element (such as tensile strength, elasticity and breaking strength)[10]	
Synthetic materials	Can be easily reconstructed into a 3D scaffold of specified microstructure, shape and dimensions [11]	Do not display the same physical properties as detrusor muscle
	Possibility of meddling with the physical properties of scaffolds (predictable physical behavior)	Lack of biological recognition (less biocompatible)
	Easier processing techniques than decellularization [12]	Do not contain cues promoting cell adhesion, proliferation and differentiation
Natural polymers	Shows minimal inflammatory and antigenic response [13]	Weak mechanical strength
	Abundant, and may be readily purified from both animal and human tissues	
	Approved by the Food and Drug Administration (FDA) for many types of medical applications [14]	Inadequate ability to tailor these biomaterials
	Less vulnerable to the enzymatic degradation [15]	A combination more than one component may not be suitable for scaffold fabrication, where only one component exhibits the required biological function [16]
	Has cell delivery and cell immobilization capability due to its gelling properties [17]	

Autologous adult derived Stem cells offer an alternative to using cells from the dysfunctional bladder. Adult stem cells are undifferentiated cells found amongst differentiated cells in different tissues and organs. They have the capacity to differentiate into cells types of different lineages and have garnered great interest in regenerative medicine due to the ethical issues with using embryonic stem cells. Adult derived stem cells including bone marrow derived and adipose derived cells have been shown to differentiate into detrusor muscle and urothelial cells and from distinct tissue layers *in vivo* consisting of urothelium, submucosa and muscle layer. Adipose derived stem cells are particularly attractive as they can potentially be harvested in larger quantities under local anaesthetic lipoaspirate biopsy.

During the culture of cells on scaffolds prior to implantation two approaches can be followed to optimize the maturing construct: addition of growth factors/cytokines or mechanical stimulation. Growth factors/cytokines are added to encourage cell growth, differentiation or to promote the production of certain extracellular matrix proteins such as elastin or collagen which convey elasticity and strength to tissues respectively. Applying a mechanical stimulus within a bioreactor, particularly one that re-creates the stresses and strains that a bladder would undergo *in vivo (i.e., filling and emptying)*, has been attempted with the aim of inducing appropriate organization of the muscle fibres and extracellular matrix proteins before implantation to improve clinical outcome [20].

Cell culture time period in the laboratory usually does not exceed 2 weeks for cell seeding on the scaffold. This is usually sufficient time for cells to reach confluence and develop extracellular matrix coverage of the scaffold. It is generally thought to be inadvisable to allow further growth as a diffusion distance of greater 3–4 mm^3 limits the gas and nutrient uptake. If cells were implanted in volumes of >3–4 mm^3 only the cells on the surface would survive, and the central cell component would be at risk of death due to lack of vascularity [21].

Vascularisation

In any reconstructive surgery a good blood supply is critical to the outcome. Thus for whole organ tissue engineering promoting angiognenesis and vasuclogenesis is paramount. Angiogenesis is the development of new vessels from pre-existing blood vessels that have been converted into an angiogenic state where as the formation of blood vessels through the *de novo* differentiation of stem cells into endothelial cells. Strategies at promoting both these processes have been attempted to increase the chance of survival of tissue-engineered constructs. Such strategies relate to the addition of pro-angiogenic factors to culture media and modification of scaffold properties to facilitate ingrowth of host cells. Perhaps the most important aspect in terms of whole bladder engineering is the time honoured surgical practice of using omentum to ensure the survival of grafts. The rich bloody supply of the omentum and its mobility is likely to make it an essential component, as was the case in the case series from Atala [3].

Innervation

Innervation is the holy grail of bladder tissue engineering and is major reason why tissue engineering for underactive bladder is not a reality in the near future. Recreating the complexities of sensory and motor innervation is beyond current capabilities in the field.

Stem Cell Injection Therapy

An alternative approach to implanting a whole engineered bladder to replace an underactive bladder, which appears a far off prospect at present, is to inject stem cells at various sites to restore bladder function. Several studies investigating different cell types to treat bladder dysfunction in animals are available. These studies follow the scheme of using a model of underactive bladder, injection of stem cells in the bladder or at site of damage to the neural innervation and then performing urodynamic assessment of bladder contractility.

Adult derived stem cells (ADSC) are considered more workable than embryonic stem cells due the ethical complexities of growing embryos for cell harvest. ADSC can be sourced from fat, bone marrow and skeletal muscle. All the cell types have similar properties in terms of differentiation and regenerative abilities. The main differences are the ease with which a tissue sample can be obtained, and how easily a population of cells can be expanded in culture. ADSC are though to exhibit a regenerative effect through migration, differentiation and a predominately a paracrine effect.

Several rodent models have been developed to study underactive bladder such as bladder outlet obstruction, cryo-injury, chronic ischaemia by bilateral iliac artery ligation, pelvic nerve injury and diabetic bladder dysfunction. Direct injection of ADSC into the bladder wall or damaged nerve lesion has resulted in some improvements contractility and bladder emptying. There is however a need for longer-term studies before protocols for pilot studies in man can be planned. The available studies are summarized in Table 11.2.

Table 11.2 Studies investigation stem cell injection therapy in underactive bladder

Study	Animal	Model	Cell type	Site of injection	Outcome
Nishijima et al. [22]	Rat	BOO	Bone marrow cells	Bladder wall	Reduction of residual urine volume and increase in contractility
Chen et al. [23]	Rat	Chronic bladder ischaemia	Bone marrow derived stem cell	Intra arterial injection	Increase in contractility
Huard et al. [24]	Mice	Cryo-injured bladder	Muscle derived cell	Bladder wall	Increase in contractility
Sakuma et al. [25]	Mice	Cryo-injured	Adipose derived stem cell	Bladder wall	Differentiation into smooth muscle cells
Nitta et al. [26]	Rat	Pelvic nerve injury	Skeletal muscle mesenchymal stem cell	Damaged nerve lesion	Increase in intravesical pressure
Kwon et al. [27]	Rat	Pelvic nerve injury	Muscle derived cell	Damaged nerve lesion	Increase intravesical pressure

Conclusion

The lack of any effective pharmacotherapy for DU/UAB has led to the consideration of whether regenerative medicine may offer solutions. Laboratory grown whole bladders have been implanted into humans for the purpose of urine storage. However the key purpose in a patient with DU/UAB would be to restore contractility and this requires a neural innervation which is beyond the reach of current technology. The alternative approach of injecting stem cells at the bladder or site of neural damage appears more workable however only small studies in animals have been performed to date. Further of investigation of this approach in man should logically ensure that stem cells are injected at a site consistent to the likely underlying cause.

References

1. Osman NI, Hillary C, Bullock AJ, MacNeil S, Chapple CR. Tissue engineered buccal mucosa for urethroplasty: progress and future directions. Adv Drug Deliv Rev. 2015;82–83:69–76. Epub 2014/12/03.
2. Tran C, Damaser MS. The potential role of stem cells in the treatment of urinary incontinence. Therapeutic advances in urology. 2015;7(1):22–40. Epub 2015/02/03.
3. Atala A, Bauer SB, Soker S, Yoo JJ, Retik AB. Tissue-engineered autologous bladders for patients needing cystoplasty. Lancet. 2006;367(9518):1241–6. Epub 2006/04/25.
4. Langer R, Vacanti JP. Tissue engineering. Science. 1993;260(5110):920–6.
5. Horst M, Madduri S, Gobet R, Sulser T, Milleret V, Hall H, et al. Engineering functional bladder tissues. J Tissue Eng Regen Med. 2013;7(7):515–22. Epub 2012/03/23.
6. Record RD, Hillegonds D, Simmons C, Tullius R, Rickey FA, Elmore D, et al. In vivo degradation of 14C-labeled small intestinal submucosa (SIS) when used for urinary bladder repair. Biomaterials. 2001;22(19):2653–9.
7. Bolland F, Korossis S, Wilshaw SP, Ingham E, Fisher J, Kearney JN, et al. Development and characterisation of a full-thickness acellular porcine bladder matrix for tissue engineering. Biomaterials. 2007;28(6):1061–70.
8. Badylak SF, Taylor D, Uygun K. Whole-organ tissue engineering: decellularization and recellularization of three-dimensional matrix scaffolds. Annu Rev Biomed Eng. 2011; 13:27–53.
9. Chen F, Yoo JJ, Atala A. Acellular collagen matrix as a possible "off the shelf" biomaterial for urethral repair. Urology. 1999;54(3):407–10. Epub 1999/09/04.
10. Aitken KJ, Bägli DJ. The bladder extracellular matrix. Part II: regenerative applications. Nat Rev Urol. 2009;6(11):612–21.
11. Choi JS, Lee SJ, Christ GJ, Atala A, Yoo JJ. The influence of electrospun aligned poly(epsilon-caprolactone)/collagen nanofiber meshes on the formation of self-aligned skeletal muscle myotubes. Biomaterials. 2008;29(19):2899–906.
12. Rim NG, Shin CS, Shin H. Current approaches to electrospun nanofibers for tissue engineering. Biomed Mater. 2013;8(1):014102.
13. Furthmayr H, Timpl R. Immunochemistry of collagens and procollagens. Int Rev Connect Tissue Res. 1976;7:61–99.
14. Cen L, Liu W, Cui L, Zhang W, Cao Y. Collagen tissue engineering: development of novel biomaterials and applications. Pediatr Res. 2008;63(5):492–6.
15. Sams AE, Nixon AJ. Chondrocyte-laden collagen scaffolds for resurfacing extensive articular cartilage defects. Osteoarthritis Cartilage. 1995;3(1):47–59.
16. Lin HK, Madihally SV, Palmer B, Frimberger D, Fung KM, Kropp BP. Biomatrices for bladder reconstruction. Adv Drug Deliv Rev. 2015;82–83:47–63.

17. Smidsrød O, Skjåk-Braek G. Alginate as immobilization matrix for cells. Trends Biotechnol. 1990;8(3):71–8.
18. Atala A. Tissue engineering of human bladder. Br Med Bull. 2011;97:81–104. Epub 2011/02/18.
19. Lai JY, Yoon CY, Yoo JJ, Wulf T, Atala A. Phenotypic and functional characterization of in vivo tissue engineered smooth muscle from normal and pathological bladders. J Urol. 2002;168(4 Pt 2):1853–7; discussion 8. Epub 2002/09/28.
20. Farhat WA, Yeger H. Does mechanical stimulation have any role in urinary bladder tissue engineering? World J Urol. 2008;26(4):301–5. Epub 2008/08/12.
21. Folkman J, Hochberg M. Self-regulation of growth in three dimensions. J Exp Med. 1973;138(4):745–53.
22. Nishijima S, Sugaya K, Miyazato M, Kadekawa K, Oshiro Y, Uchida A, et al. Restoration of bladder contraction by bone marrow transplantation in rats with underactive bladder. Biomed Res. 2007;28(5):275–80. Epub 2007/11/15.
23. Chen S, Zhang HY, Zhang N, Li WH, Shan H, Liu K, et al. Treatment for chronic ischaemia-induced bladder detrusor dysfunction using bone marrow mesenchymal stem cells: an experimental study. Int J Mol Med. 2012;29(3):416–22. Epub 2011/11/24.
24. Huard J, et al. Muscle-derived cell-mediated ex vivo gene therapy for urological dysfunction. Gene Ther. 2002;9(23):1617–26.
25. Sakuma T, Matsumoto T, Kano K, Fukuda N, Obinata D, Yamaguchi K, et al. Mature, adipocyte derived, dedifferentiated fat cells can differentiate into smooth muscle-like cells and contribute to bladder tissue regeneration. J Urol. 2009;182(1):355–65. Epub 2009/05/22.
26. Nitta M, Tamaki T, Tono K, Okada Y, Masuda M, Akatsuka A, et al. Reconstitution of experimental neurogenic bladder dysfunction using skeletal muscle-derived multipotent stem cells. Transplantation. 2010;89(9):1043–9. Epub 2010/02/13.
27. Kwon D, Minnery B, Kim Y, Kim JH, de Miguel F, Yoshimura N, et al. Neurologic recovery and improved detrusor contractility using muscle-derived cells in rat model of unilateral pelvic nerve transection. Urology. 2005;65(6):1249–53. Epub 2005/06/01.

Reflections and the Way Forward

12

Nadir I. Osman, Chistopher R. Chapple, and Alan J. Wein

The last two decades in urology has seen major refinements in thought with regards to the categorization of lower urinary tracts symptoms (LUTS) and the understanding of the underlying pathophysiological basis of these symptoms. For the most part there has been an overwhelming focus on detrusor overactivity (DO) and bladder outlet obstruction (BOO) as the causes storage and voiding LUTS respectively. This focus has been beneficial in that it has generated a large body of basic and clinical research that has furthered our understanding and led to the development of numerous beneficial medical and surgical therapies. By contrast the problem of detrusor underactivity (DU), although recognized, has been largely neglected and it is salutary to note that last major advance in management was the introduction of clean intermittent catheterization by Jack Lapides over 40 years ago.

In the last 5 years there has been resurgence in interest in DU with efforts having been initiated to better define the problem, understand it epidemiology, aetiology and pathogenesis with a view to developing new treatments that may benefit patients. The problem of definition is challenging, the International continence society (ICS) has a definition for DU, a urodynamic diagnosis, which is conceptual rather than prescriptive. The definition lacks detail on what constitutes reduced contraction strength and length which hampers its practical application. There is certainly a need for further refinement of this definition which will need to be directed by focus group studies of both healthy individuals and those with symptom evaluated with

N.I. Osman
Urology SpR, The Royal Hallamshire Hospital, Sheffield, South Yorkshire, UK
e-mail: nadirosman@hotmail.com

C.R. Chapple
Department of Urology, The Royal Hallamshire Hospital, Sheffield, UK
e-mail: c.r.chapple@shef.ac.uk

A.J. Wein (✉)
Urology, Perelman Center, West Pavilion, 3rd Floor, Philadelphia, PA, USA
e-mail: alan.wein@uphs.upenn.edu

C.R. Chapple et al. (eds.), *Underactive Bladder*,
DOI 10.1007/978-3-319-43087-4_12

urodynamic investigation to provide the best symptom/functional correlations. From the epidemiological perspective it is clear that our understanding is very limited. The need for a urodynamic study to establish the urodynamic diagnosis has prevented the acquisition of any population data. Clinical urodynamic series have been used as a surrogate, which have shown the surprisingly common occurrence of DU in both men and women. However it is important to temper this finding with the fact that these groups studied are in fact 'patients' with refractory LUTS being seen in secondary care which introduces a significant degree of selection bias. Nevertheless DU appears to be sufficiently common in the group of patients seen in urological practice to warrant further study on a population basis, as it does appear to be an important condition affecting the population which increases in prevalence with increasing age.

To better understand the epidemiology, it worthwhile to draw the analogy to the problem of detrusor overactivity (DO)- the urodynamic diagnosis and overactive bladder (OAB)-the symptom complex. The latter has helped us to better understand the prevalence of the underlying bladder, dysfunction albeit the two are variably correlated. A similar approach could potentially be taken with detrusor underactivity (DU) – again the urodynamic diagnosis and the underactive bladder (UAB) its associated symptoms. The symptom complex of UAB is an emerging concept that is generating great interest at present, not only for its value from an epidemiological perspective but because it could allow the diagnosis and potential initiation of treatment without the need for invasive urodynamic investigation, which is of course not feasible in primary care.

The working definition of UAB which has been proposed is a good starting point; but the major concern is that it will not be able to sufficiently differentiate those patients with DU from those whose symptoms have arisen secondary to BOO or even DO, since the symptoms of OAB overlap with many of those seen in UAB. To improve the specificity of the definition there is need for prospective quantitative studies as well as qualitative studies to better understand the symptoms that characterize DU. Such studies are now underway. Ultimately it may also be necessary to add some form of objective non-invasive test to achieve acceptable specificity in diagnosis. It is apparent that an easily implemented non expensive tests is not currently available, in this respect ultrasonic measurement of detrusor wall thickness and penile cuff urodynamics are worthy of further evaluation and validation. In addition further evaluation of newer technologies, eg near infrared spectroscopy which has failed to find a substantive role to date could be promising.

Though invasive urodynamics form the cornerstone of the diagnosis of DU, there is a remarkable lack of clarity on which is the best method. The bladder outlet relation as described by Derek Griffiths, forms the basis of most methods to estimate bladder contraction strength, such as the bladder contractility index and stop tests. However it is clear that contraction strength is only one aspect normal detrusor contraction, the others being speed, sustainability and coordination of a detrusor contraction. At present we have no reliable method to estimate the relative importance of these individual aspects as such they have been formally evaluated in only a few studies. It is also important to remember the central role an intact bladder sensation plays in the micturition reflex and it would be helpful for future studies investigation diagnostic criteria to include this aspect, into the complex evaluation process.

The aetiopathogenesis of DU is likely to be multifactorial as we can clearly see that wide range diseases and injuries can be manifest as DU. Itemising the components potentially involved in DU and the UAB symptom complex, the site of underlying pathophysiology is either the detrusor muscle itself, the innervation (sensory or motor) or the central coordination of neural signals. The lack of epidemiological data makes it difficult to understand the common aetiologies or indeed natural history of the condition. Despite a common perception as noted above. It is by no means firmly established that normal ageing or bladder obstruction are the primary causes.

Effective pharmacotherapy for the treatment of DU/UAB is currently not available. The most commonly studied class to date are the parasympathomimetics, the efficacy of which cannot be supported by the available evidence. There is certainly a need for further studies and the development of new agents. The major issue is that bladder emptying represents only 1 % of micturition cycle and the risk of side effects of any new agent should be balanced against this. In addition, if bladder innervation is disturbed i.e. a problem of impaired sensory function, then an agent which aims to increase contractility may still be ineffective and may indeed result in dysfunctional bladder behavior which is not advantageous. Ultimately there is need to develop a better understanding of the mechanism involved in the generation of normal voiding contraction and common defects in those with DU, to better target drug development.

Surgical therapies have shown limited success in treating DU. In men with DU who are dependent on catheters many surgeons would advocated de obstructive surgery provided the patient is fit, however success rates are clearly lower than in those with preserved contractility. We do not feel there is any role for bladder outlet surgery in women with DU due to the risks of incontinence due to damage to the sphincteric mechanism. Bladder reconstruction to reduced bladder capacity has very limited evidence to support it and seldom practiced in contemporary times. At other end of the spectrum bladder myoplasty surgery has shown promising results, however the scale complexity and invasiveness of the surgery are unlikely to result in widespread application given the availability of clean intermittent catheterization. In addition this is complex surgery which has only been conducted in a very highly selected group of patients and is not without morbidity. Electrical stimulation techniques are more likely to be acceptable to patients and clinicians however the evidence for their efficacy outside specific neurogenic situations is limited, but warrants further exploration.

In conclusion, the problems of DU and it symptom correlate UAB present a major challenge to the clinical and scientific communities. There is need for a concerted effort to be made to improve our knowledge and understanding of almost all aspects of this problem. With increasing recognition of DU/UAB we hope that in the future progress toward developing safe and effective treatments will be made.

Index

C.R. Chapple et al. (eds.), *Underactive Bladder*,
DOI 10.1007/978-3-319-43087-4

MIX
Papier aus verantwortungsvollen Quellen
Paper from responsible sources
FSC® C105338

If you have any concerns about our products,
you can contact us on
ProductSafety@springernature.com

In case Publisher is established outside the EU,
the EU authorized representative is:
Springer Nature Customer Service Center GmbH
Europaplatz 3, 69115 Heidelberg, Germany

Printed by Libri Plureos GmbH
in Hamburg, Germany